THE RE-CENTER METHOD NATURAL DIET

SOUP BOOK

Celebrate the Joy of Soups International Recipes from 7 Continents to boast your metabolism in Just 8 weeks

Hareldau Argyle King

Also Available from Refinement Publishing & Media

Quotes to Habits
Remember
Hareldau Argyle King

The Re-center Method
Natural Diet
Hareldau Argyle King

The Re-center Method
Natural Diet Cookbook
Hareldau Argyle King

Web site: www.beingelevatedlifestyle.com
Email: support@beingelevatedlifestyle.com

As with all exercises and dietary programs, you should get your doctor's approval before beginning. The information here is to help you make an informed decision about your health.

This book is not intended as a substitute for any treatment that may have been prescribed by your doctor. The reader should regularly consult a doctor in matters about his/her health and particularly concerning any symptoms that may require diagnosis or medical attention.

This book is intended as a reference manual and not a medical manual. The exercises and dietary programs in the book are not intended as a substitute for any exercise routine or dietary regimen that may have been prescribed by your doctor.

www.beingelevatedlifestyle.com
ISBN 978-1-950838-30-1 - Ebook
ISBN: 978-1-950838-31-8- Paperback
ISBN: 978-1-950838-32-5- Hardback

ACKNOWLEDGMENTS

Meals taste better when shared in the community, and even better when shared with stories among family, friends, and colleagues.

I am grateful for every friend, family member, and & passing acquaintance I shared a unique meal, whether the meals were a local dish or an elaborate international meal.

Whether it was served at a dinner party, upscale restaurant, a local diner, or a backyard cookout. In every city I lived, town I passed through, and country every visited I say Thank you.

Your generosity encouraged me to gather & create this collection of recipes from different states and nations.

FOREWORD

When I was 20 years old, I sought out Hareldau–who was a world-renowned athlete– to get me in peak performance. She was my fitness coach for a beauty pageant and later coached me when I went to the nationals. Hareldau is an outstanding leader and through the course of her fitness coaching, she became my life coach, my mentor, and my friend.

Had it not been for her coaching and guidance, I would not have honed my voice as a public speaker and communicator nor been crowned Miss District of Columbia Sweetheart 2015 in my very first beauty pageant. Hareldau's guidance in business, fitness and in life has had a huge impact on my path as a professional, creative, and finally, as a person.

Hareldau's commitment to health and well-being is reflected in her talent for helping others learn how to nourish themselves. Her focus on a well-rounded and eclectic diet through international cooking is a diverse methodology to incentivizing fitness and wellness in such a way that we can view our diet through the lens of lifestyle– from our food choices to our thoughts.

As readers matriculate through each region of the world, I advise them to read the excerpts that give us glimpses of information about each locale so that they are able to experience these recipes to their fullest while expanding their breadth of understanding.

This approach to health and wellness reflects Hareldau's appreciation for all the world's culinary facets and why each of us can feel encouraged–not only to view health in a more wholesome and exciting way– but to nourish ourselves, body and mind, through the richness and cultural diversity that is just beyond our doorstep!

Through each of these keepsake recipes, we can learn how to improve our diets in a new way while developing a cultural appreciation for every region of the world and expanding our taste palettes simultaneously.

It is my most earnest wish that readers and food connoisseurs experience the richness of culinary diversity, the profound impact of nourishing your overall health by loving what's in your bowl, the health and wellness benefits of each of these 52 international recipes, and the excitement of traveling within your own home.

I have never known a more determined, brilliant, and dynamic healer with such an incredible capacity for not only understanding others of every walk of life through compassion, but for helping others thrive in all aspects of their lives: peak fitness, confidence, emotional well-being, leadership and last but certainly not least, through healthy eating—all through deliberate action, nurturing, and lifestyle improvement.

Without further ado, it is my deepest honor to highly recommend Hareldau as a fitness and health specialist, a life coach, a public speaker, a thought leader, a traveler, and a cultural enthusiast, and finally, as a cook and an author.

May these recipes from all corners of the globe inspire readers to travel within the comfort of their homes and to nourish their bodies, minds, and souls by embracing delightful foods from around the world.

Sydney Hall
Miss District of Columbia Sweetheart 2015

DEDICATION

IN HONOR OF
SYDNEY ALEXIS HALL

In honor of my friend, mentee, and humanitarian
Ms. Sydney Alexis Halls lives a life of adventure, justice &possibilities
You are a source of joy, artistry & constant growth
A kindred soul, beautiful spirit, a caring friend
Your daringness to take on new challenges, live in different countries, and face obstacles head-on is breathtaking
You wear your heart for justice, equality, and diversity on your sleeves
You are irreplaceable!

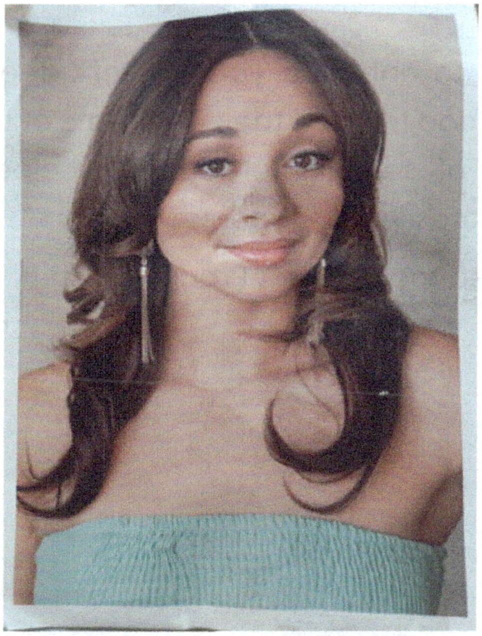

Sydney Alexis Hall

How to Use this Book

This book is a guide to a higher quality of life, through building relationships and varying your food choices. Whether you never had an international meal or friend or whether this is your way of life, there are words of encouragement, new ideas & solutions to enhance your quality of life.

The book is divided into 4 sections. The first section is seasonal Soups recipes from North America -fall, winter, spring & summer.

Section 11 consists of breakfast recipes, Section 111 Lunch recipes, and section 1v dinner recipes from 7 continents. If you notice a country under a different classification, it may be because some countries may be geographically located in one continent as well as cultural associate with another.

This is not a diet book, a weight loss book, or a meal plan. On your first attempt to prepare these dishes, your meal may or may not look like the photo of the meal in this book.

This book is designed to enhance your tastebud, exposing you to different textures and tastes of food from all the continents of the world. After you would complete this 4-part of series international recipe books you experience cuisines from 195 countries in 7 continents.

I invite you to get started today. Don't Procrastinate!!

Table of Content

Table of Content

Table of Content

Table of Content

Table of Content

Introduction

Dear Friend,

Celebrating the joy of healthy eating of global cuisine is essential for a sustainable lifestyle.

When was the last time you had a new food experience? Cooked a new healthy meal, dined at different exotic international restaurants, or shopped at a specialty supermarket?

Embracing different textures, types, and touches of food adds to living a full, fit, and fun lifestyle.

It is often said that books you read or don't read reflect your mindset, your bank, and your credit card statement since reflecting your priorities and what you value. Glancing into your shopping basket at the grocery store or farmer's market reflects your waistline, your taste bud, and your food tendencies.

As a fitness professional, nutrition specialist, and food & culture enthusiast, I am constantly observing other people's food habits in grocery stores and restaurants while managing my own. I find myself curiously observing other people's shopping habits in the checkout aisle, much the way friends and family come over to examine what's on my plate and in glass at a cocktail or dinner party. A wiser statement a friend said to me about food choices is "every time I do grocery shopping, I purchase at least one item I have never tried before" This statement inspires me every day.

A glance into your shopping cart will tell me where you spend most of your time shopping and the quality of the food you are buying, whether it is in between the aisle getting lots of cans, frozen meals, and bagged snacks or on the perimeter of the store getting fresh fruits & vegetables, lean cuts of meats or you explored the international aisle add some variety to your healthy meals.

In college is where my love language of international cuisines & curiosities started. I went to school with students from many nations while sticking to a healthy southern meal plan of cafeteria food for track athletes and surviving the tortuous bayou heat. I was starting to desire geera, masala, curry, jerk, and other tantalizing flavors.

I intentionally started seeking out international students making new friends and embracing new cultures. It was my low-budget way of gathering recipes, tasting new cuisines, and sharing stories about the uniqueness of culture from people from around the world. I quickly discovered almost every culture has a unique way of preparing two things: bread and rice & peas.

I was intentional about making new friends, I think I met and had a friend from almost every nation that was represented on the LSU campus. I can still remember the taste, the stories shared, and many friends as we connected over meals. We didn't have many resources, and we didn't have much time, yet we found a way to tear down walls of isolation and build bridges with each other through food and stories about family and traditions.

This book is a continuation of the food experiences that have profoundly changed and shaped my lifestyle. This collection of recipes gathered is in a 4-part series. Part 1 – Cookbook, part 2- A Soup book, part 3- Salad book, and Part 4 Smoothie book a total of 195 countries that will be released over 12 months period. It is a gift I have been given in college I now give to you.

Have you ever wondered how unpleasant life would be without good food? Food is an essential requirement for growth and tissue repair. It's equally important that you make nutritious food choices.

It has been proposed that breakfast is the most important food for the day. A healthy choice is another factor. Better breakfast options include a mix of protein, healthy fat, and fiber with little or no added sugar. The food eaten upon waking is used to refuel the body after a prolonged night of fasting and sets the pace for the rest of the day.

Each meal in the day is important to attain and sustain a healthy lifestyle. Research shows that people who eat breakfast have lesser consumption of calories throughout the day, are more likely to gain healthier muscle weight, and are less likely to experience morning fatigue and emotional instabilities.

Lunch is another important part of a day's meal. This is because eating in the afternoon replenishes the depleted energy reserves to enable you to regain focus through the activities of the day. It also supplies glucose to the blood for healthy brain function.

Dinner completes the daily food intake that may be inadequate during the day. Dinner must be also nutritious and lean; to help prepare the body that is going resting stage for a good night's sleep and recovery.

A lifestyle of healthy living is a celebration of healthy eating. Food is good its purpose is to fuel the body with energy to do work, work in the gym or the field, work in the office or at home. Food is also used as a connector, whether among friends at school in the cafeteria or colleagues at lunch in the office, or among families at dinner.

This cookbook consists of 54 recipes for soupsfor breakfast, lunch, and dinner.

I invite you to explore each continent and all the nations. That exploration journey starts in this cookbook, and leads to the international aisle in the supermarket, on towards your table and table bud. The ultimate hope is that this new healthy food experience would lead to purchasing a ticket to visit a nation, build connections and make new friends along the way. If for some reason you are unable to travel to another country because of time, money, safety, or the borders are chosen because of a health crisis. You still have an opportunity to experience a new food experience, a new way of eating, and a new way of living through the pages of this book. The Re-center Method Natural Diet Soup book

Celebrating the joy of healthy eating of global cuisine is essential for a sustainable lifestyle.

Joyfully

Hareldau Argyle King

Founder of Being Elevated Lifestyle

SECTION 1

SEASONAL SOUPS OF NORTH AMERICA

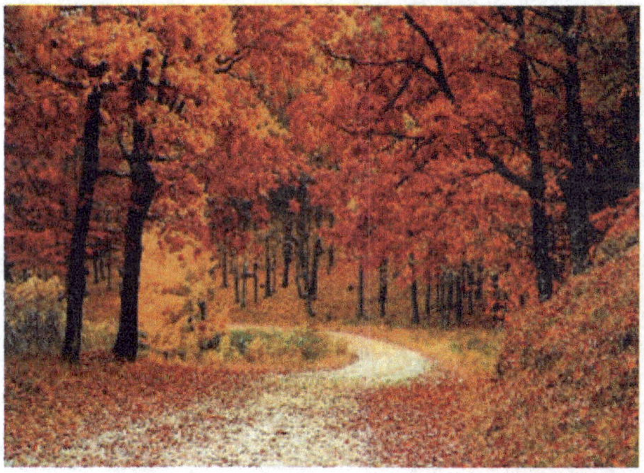
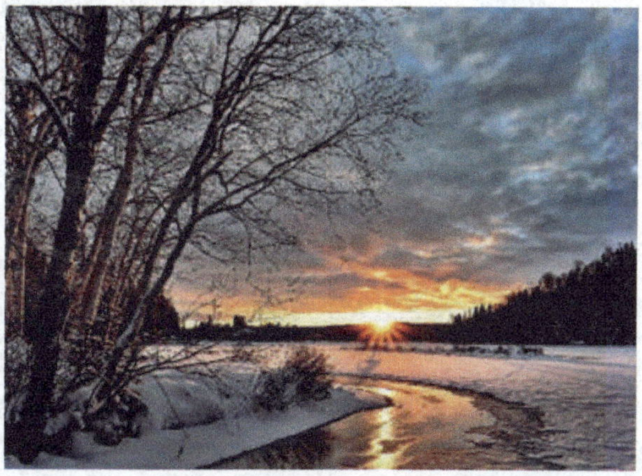
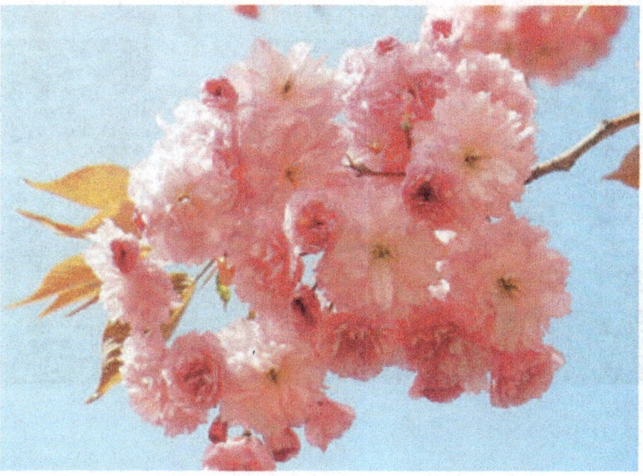
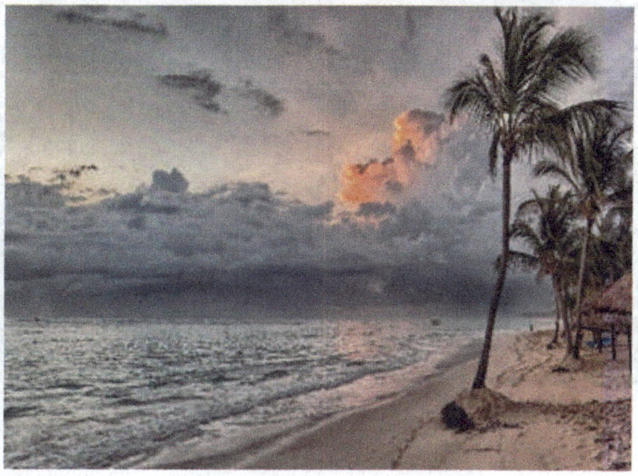

FALL SOUPS

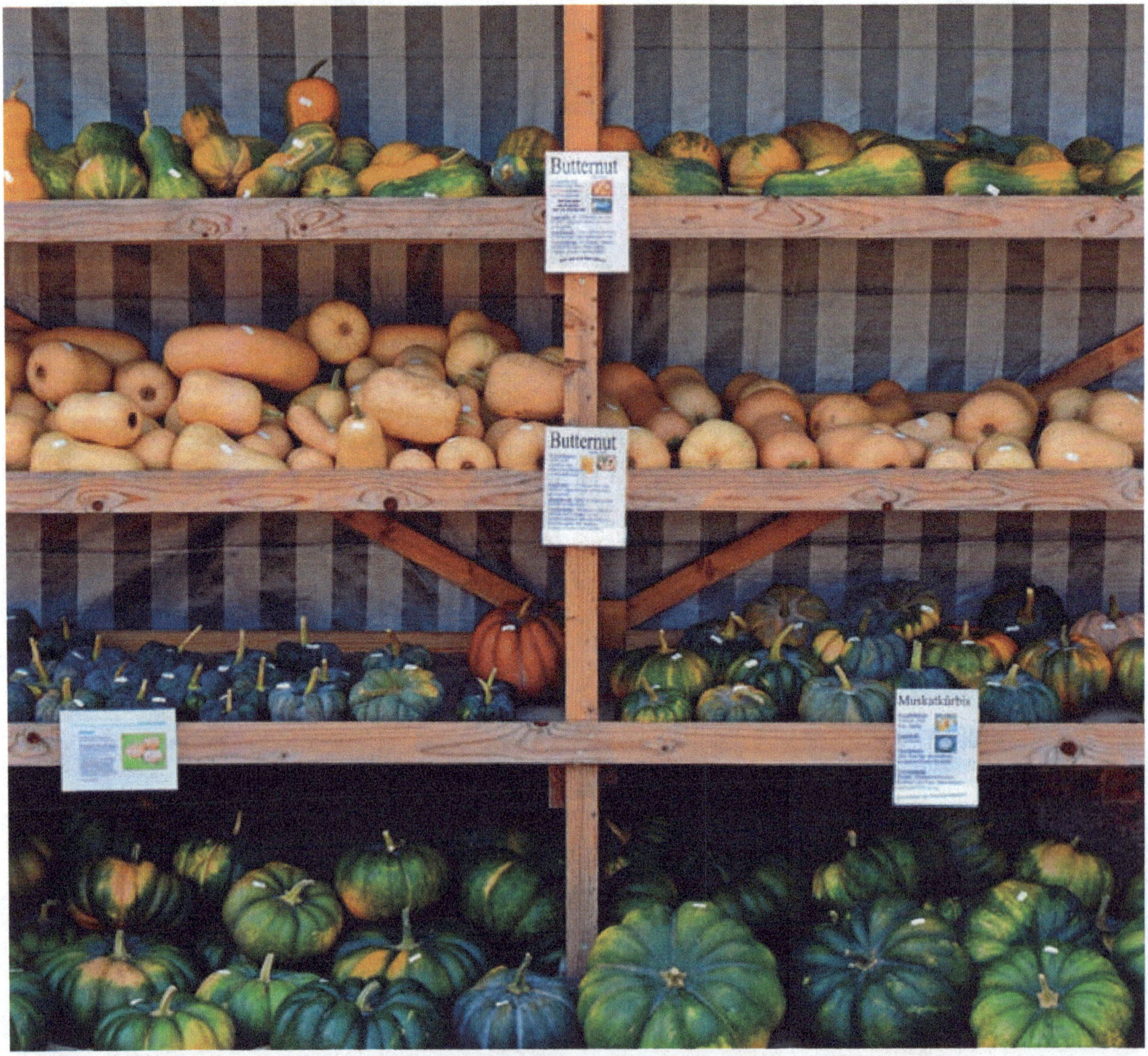

GREENLAND

Greenland is the largest island nation recorded. Glaciers and robust tundra arepart of this Arctic nation. The beautiful pre-historic culture and origin of Greenland hold much relevance to date. Its capital region is Nuuk.An average Greenlandic diet is largely meaty or marine-life based. It is challengingto grow vegetables.

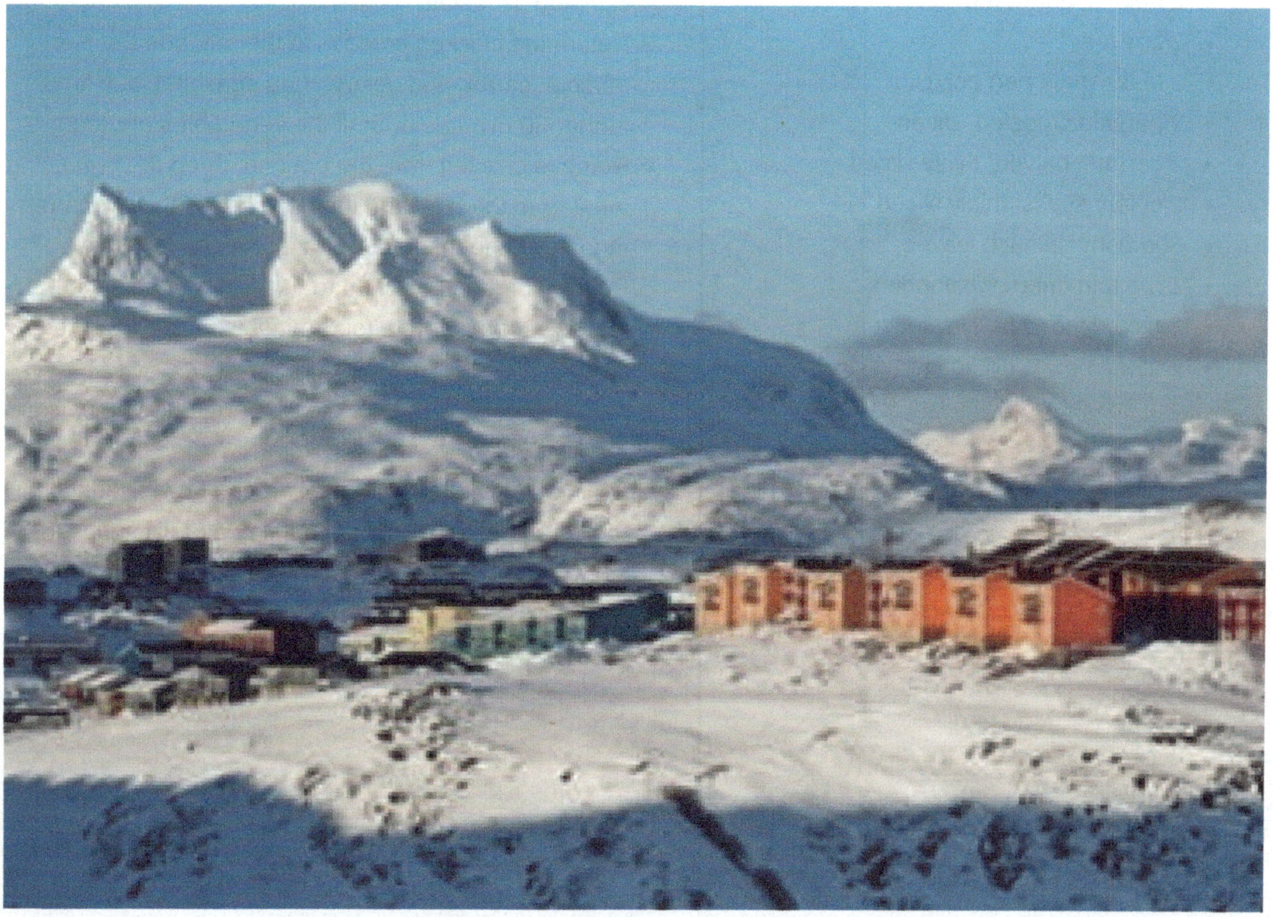

Chicken Noodle Soup

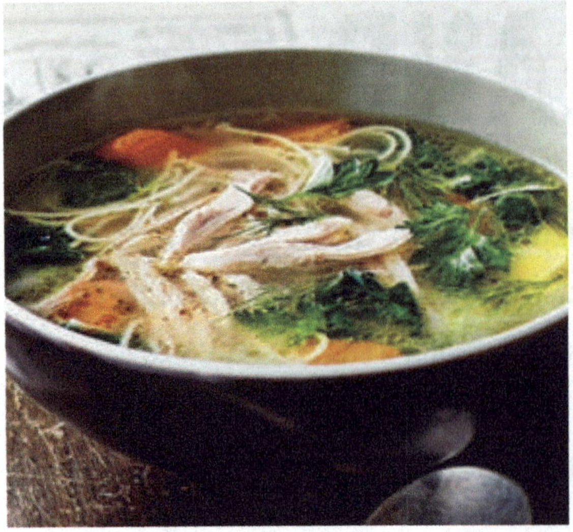

The best thing that can happen during fall is this yummy soup. There's nothing better than a bowl of golden chicken broth with root vegetables and herbsall be made in one pot.

INGREDIENTS

- 1.6kg whole chicken
- 2 onions, quartered
- 2 bay leaves
- 2 leeks (pale part only)
- 2 parsnips, peeled, sliced
- 2 carrots, halved, thinly sliced
- 2 celery stalks, thinly sliced
- 50g baby spinach leaves
- 170g thin dried egg noodles
- 2 tablespoons parsley leaves
- 2 tablespoons dill sprigs

DIRECTIONS

1. Rinse chicken and pat dry with paper towel. Place in a large stockpot and add 2 1/2L (10 cups) cold water. Add onion and bay leaves (top with a saucer to keep chicken submerged). Bring to a boil over medium-high heat. Reduce heat to medium and cook, skimming impurities from the surface, for 30 minutes or until cooked through.
2. Remove chicken from pan. Carve off the breast fillets on either side of the breastbone, remove and discard skin and set aside.
3. Return the chicken carcass to the pot, add the leek, parsnip, carrot, and celery, then season. Cook for a further 30 minutes or until the vegetables are tender.
4. Remove chicken from the pot and shred the remaining meat from the legs and thighs, discarding skin. Shred meat from the reserved breast fillets.
5. Return shredded chicken to the pan with spinach leaves. Cook, stirring, for 5 minutes or until warmed through.
6. Meanwhile, cook the noodles according to the packet instructions.
7. Drain and divide the noodles among bowls, ladle over the soup,then garnish with parsley and dill sprigs to serve.

NORTH CAROLINA, USA

The southeastern region of the United Stateshas its capital in Raleigh.

Lovers of Barbecue will love it in this region with a population of over 10,678,831 people.

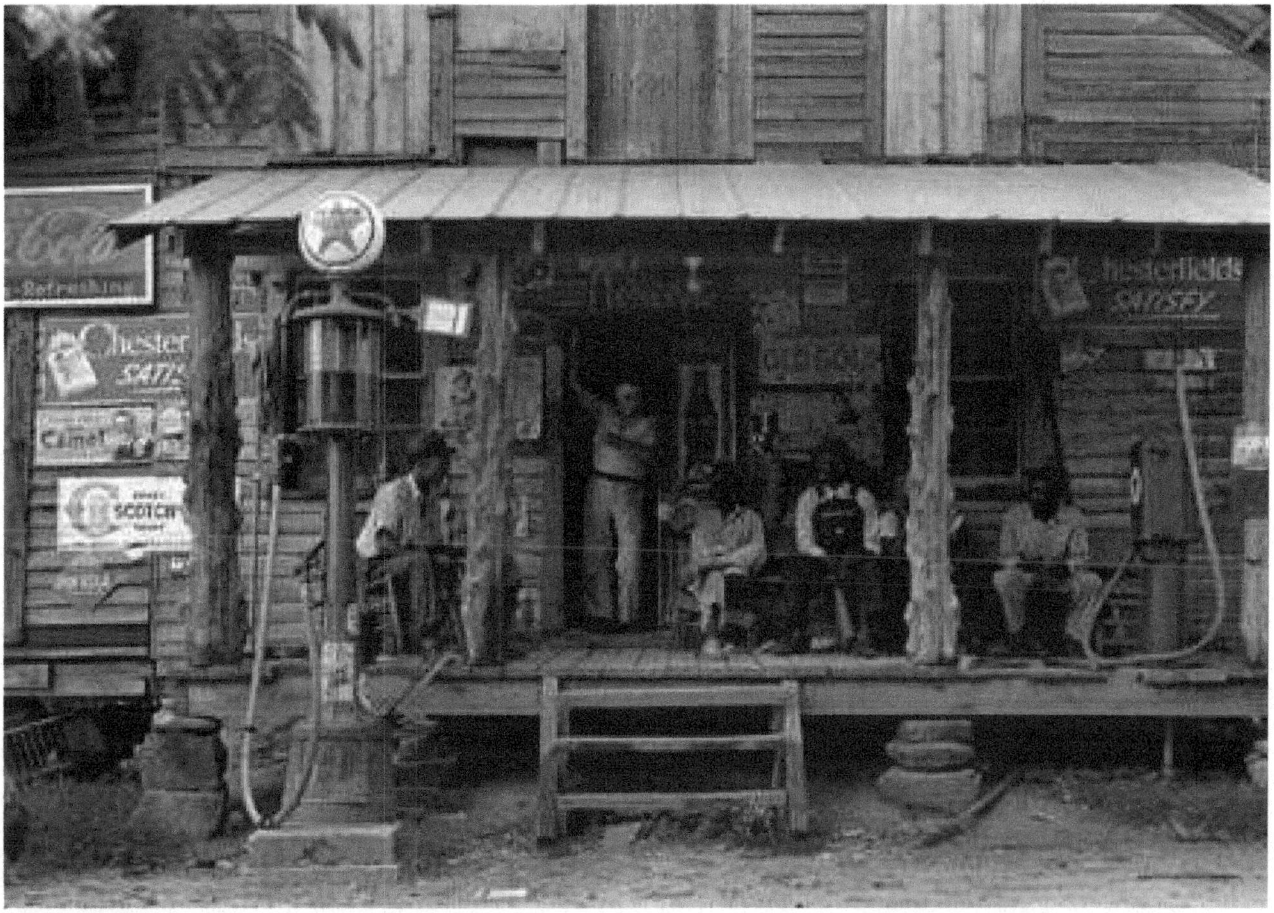

Recipe Spicy Four-Onion Soup

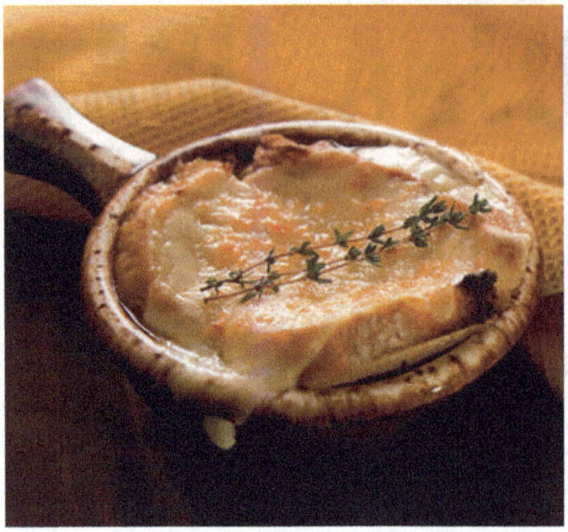

This comforting spicy goodness was designed to warm you up during fall. Four varieties of onions; red, white, yellow, and green were used in making this North Carolina delicacy.

INGREDIENTS

- 2 tablespoons butter
- 2 tablespoons olive oil
- 2 yellow onions, sliced
- 2 red onions, sliced
- 2 white onions, sliced
- 2 cloves garlic, minced
- 8 cups beef stock
- 1 cup white wine
- 2 bay leaves
- 1 sprig fresh thyme (or ½ teaspoon dried)
- salt and pepper, to taste
- 6 slices French bread, ½-inch thick, toasted and lightly buttered
- 2 cups torn cheese
- ½ cup minced Parmesan cheese
- ½ cup green onions, sliced
- Can substitute 2 tablespoons of balsamic vinegar and 2 tablespoons of brown sugar for wine

DIRECTIONS

1. In a large saucepan, heat butter and oil. Add onions, stirring occasionally, until they are very soft and lightly browned, about 1 hour. Add garlic and stir until fragrant.
2. Add beef stock, wine, bay leaves, thyme, and salt and pepper to taste. Allow flavors to meld over low heat for about 2 hours.
3. To serve, ladle soup into oven-safe bowls, topping each with a piece of toasted French bread. Evenly distribute the cheese onto the bread.
4. Set bowls on a baking sheet, and place under the broiler. Watching carefully, broil until cheese is light brown and bubbly. Remove from oven, and garnish with green onions. Serve immediately.

The best of the fall season is savored with a glass of spice apple cranberry rum punch whilst you experience Asheville.

MEXICO CITY, MEXICO

Mexico City has s a lot of importance to North America, it is the largest city, as well as the largest town.It isthe official state capital of Mexico.

The city has the largest population of Spanish-speaking people. The current population has been estimated as 131,100,519.

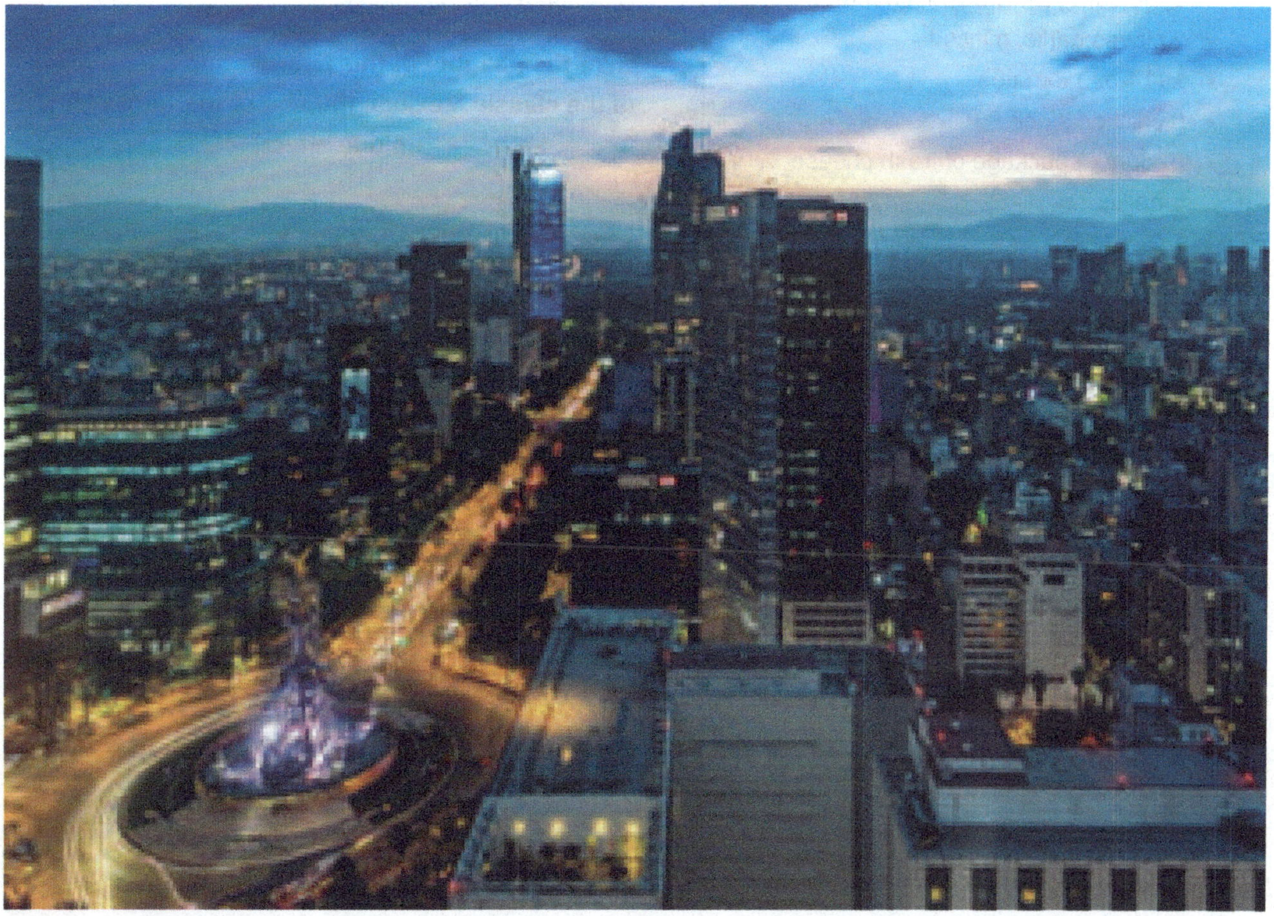

Chicken-and-Spinach Tortellini Soup

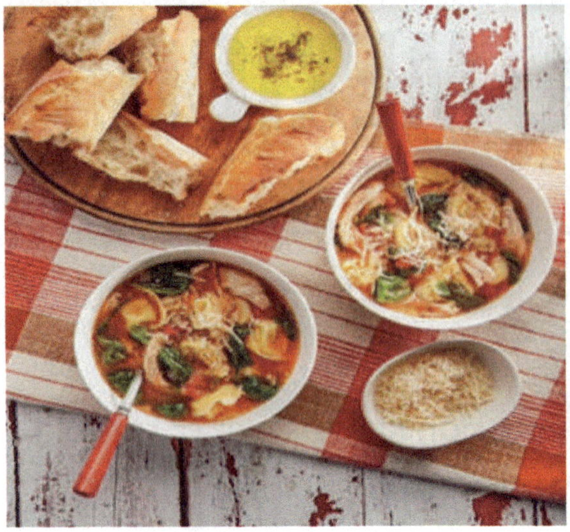

This warm bunch of goodness can be prepared in 30 minutes. It is a great warm-you—up option during fall for busy cooks.

INGREDIENTS

- 1 tbsp. olive oil
- 1 medium yellow onion, chopped
- 2 cloves garlic, minced
- 1 (14-oz.) tomatoes
- 6 chicken stock
- (9-ounce) package of fresh cheese tortellini
- 1 (5-ounce) fresh spinach
- 1/2 rotisserie chicken, shredded (about 10 ounces)
- 1/2 to 1 teaspoon crushed red pepper
- 1 tbsp. fresh lemon juice
- Grated Parmesan, torn basil leaves, and pesto, for serving

DIRECTIONS

1. Heat oil in a large pot over medium heat, Add onion and cook, stirring occasionally, until softened, 5 to 7 minutes. Add garlic and cook, stirring occasionally, until fragrant, 1 to 2 minutes. Add tomatoes and stock. Bring to a boil over high heat. Reduce to a simmer and cook 5 to 6 minutes.
2. Add tortellini and cook for 5 minutes. Add spinach and cook until wilted, 4 to 5 minutes. Reduce heat to low and add chicken, red pepper, and lemon juice. Cook until warm, 1 to 2 minutes. Serve immediately garnished with Parmesan.

Savor the delights of this hearty soup over a glass of the classic Mexican Paloma or margarita for a unique effect!

NOVA SCOTIA, CANADA

Nova Scotia means 'New Scotland' in Latin. It is a part of the thirteen provinces of Canada, in North America. It has a current population of over 1.5 million people and its capital city is Halifax Regional Municipality.

Pristine lighthouses, Abundant apples/blueberries, and robust marine life are just a bit of this province. Seafood lovers will miss out completely if Lunenberg (the lobster house) is not visited!

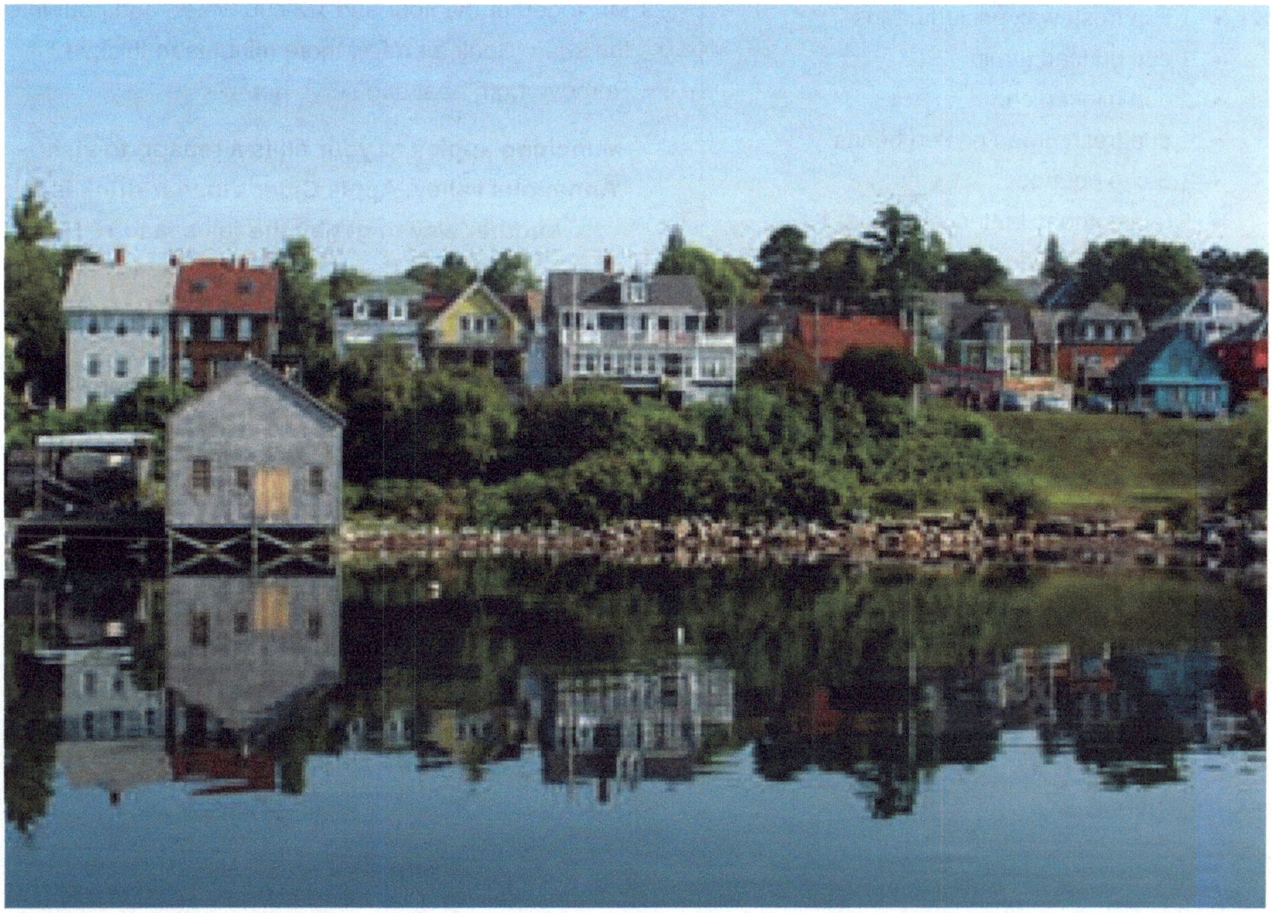

Recipe Nova Scotian Hodge Podge

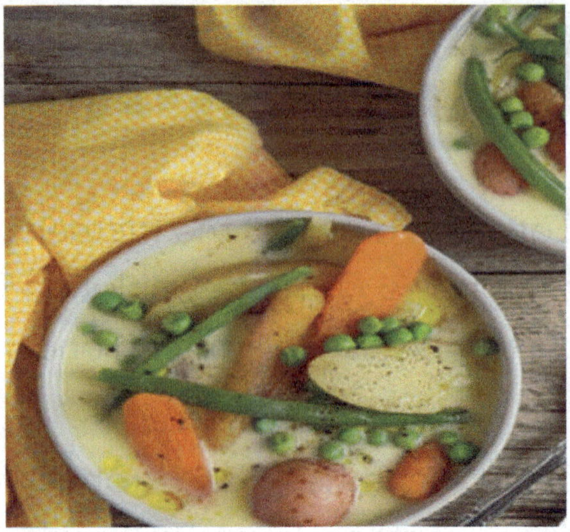

Amount of calories per serving is 241.

INGREDIENTS

- 1 cup fresh wax peeled beans
- 1 cup minced turnip
- 1 cup minced carrot
- 1 cup fresh green peeled beans
- 1.5 cup potatoes
- 5 tablespoons butter
- 1.5 cup whipped cream
- I tbsp flour
- 1.5 glass of water

This is an old favorite vegetable stew from Nova Scotia.
It is typically made in the fall as gardens are just harvested.
It is important that the freshest veggies are used.
Vary the amount by adding different vegetables and quantities.

DIRECTIONS

1. Place the green beans, wax beans, carrots, and turnips into a saucepan and add enough water to cover the vegetables.
2. Lightly salt the water and bring it to a boil. Cook for about 1/2 hour, then add the potatoes and cook for another 1/2 hour. Stir in butter and if desired, cream.
3. Mix together the flour and 1/2 cup water, and pour into the soup. Cook for a few more minutes to thicken. Remove from heat and serve hot.

Munching apples to your fill is a reason to visit Annapolis valley. Apple Cider Vinegar drink is another way to get by the fall season

WINTER SOUPS

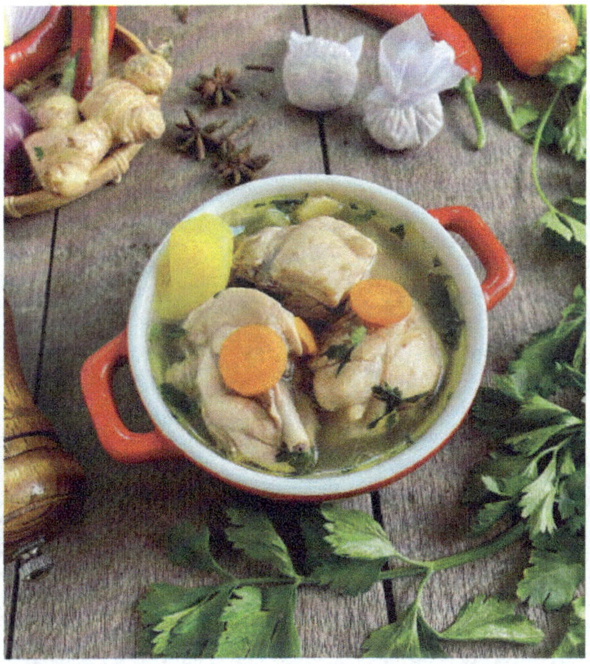

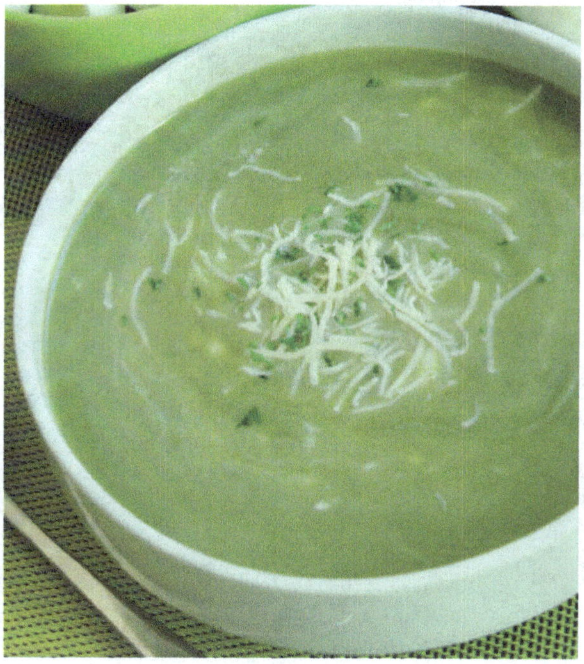

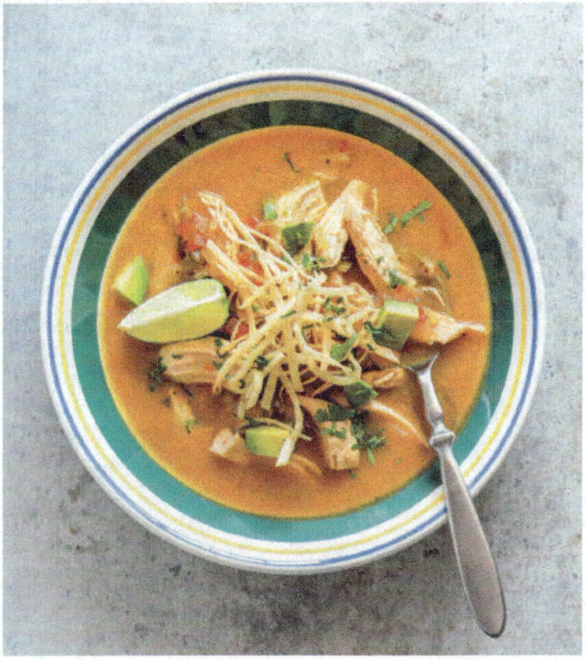

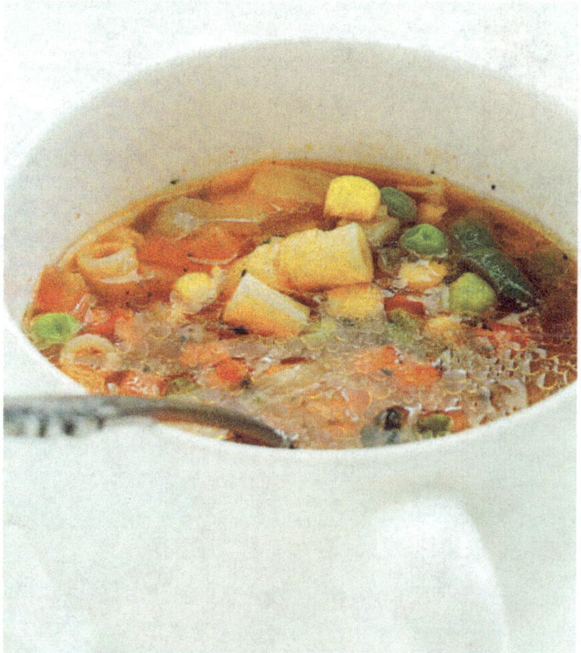

GREENLAND

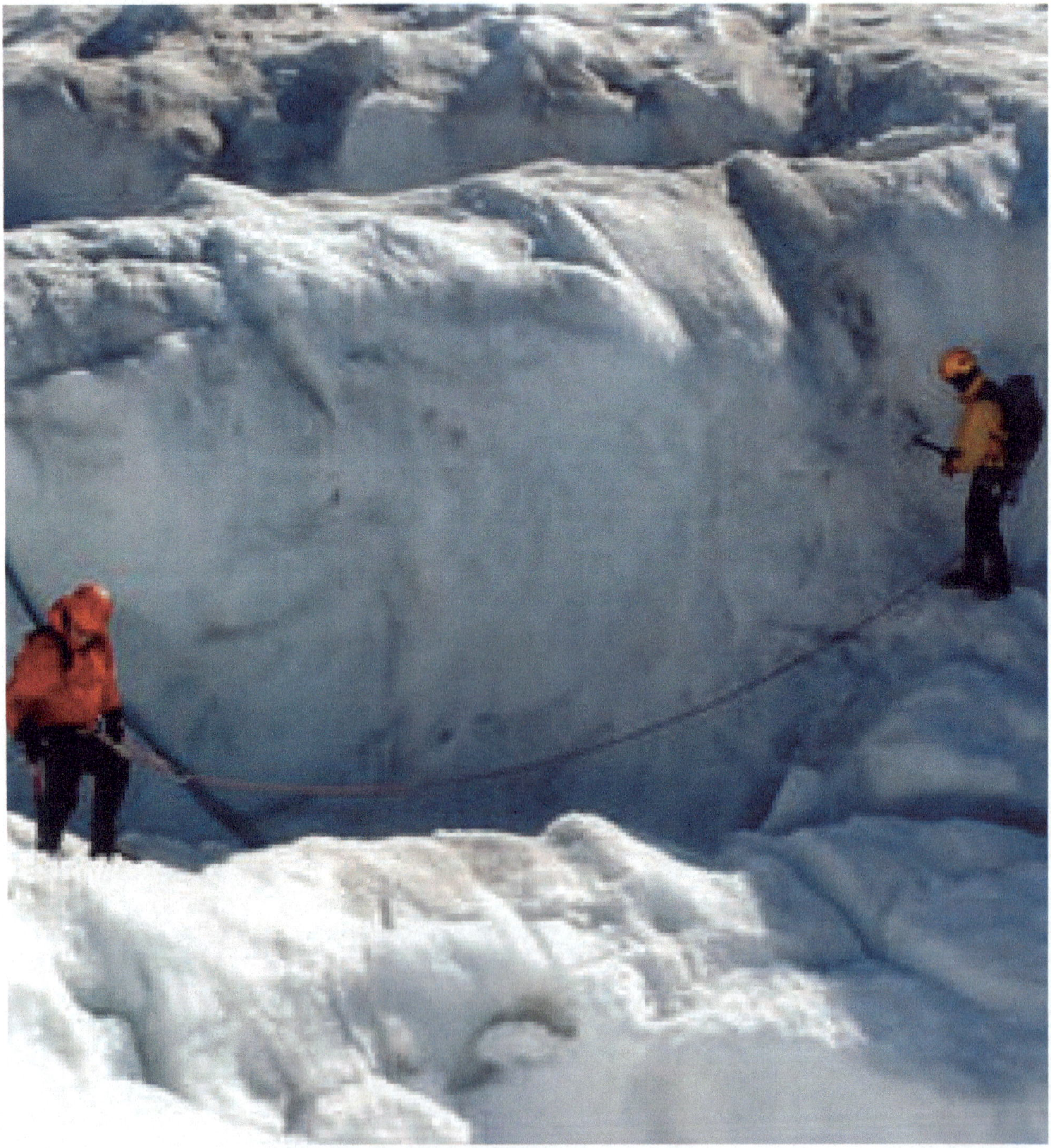

Winter Green Soup

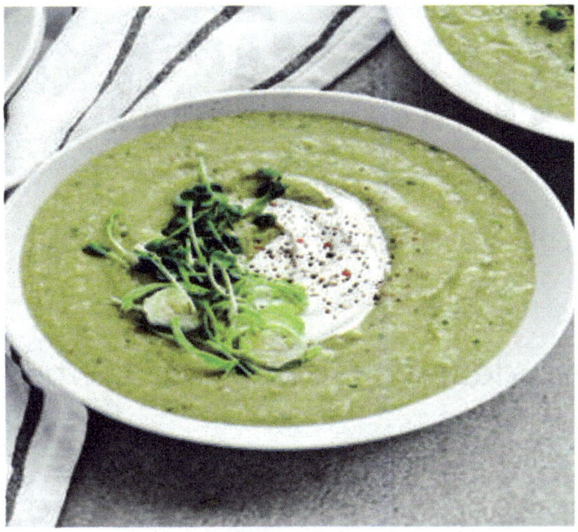

This nourishing Winter Green Soup is the perfect warmer for the cooler months with kale, broccoli, and spinach.This recipe is sure to boost your immunity.

Wintergreen soup is low carb, packed with cruciferous vegetables (broccoli, cauliflower, Brussels, etc.)

Each serving contains 29 Calories.

INGREDIENTS

- ¼ cup olive oil
- 1 large onion, peeled, sliced
- 4 cloves garlic, peeled
- 6 stalks of celery
- 2 carrots, peeled, diced
- 150g brown basmati rice
- 1 teaspoon ground cumin
- 1 teaspoon mixed spice
- ¼ teaspoon freshly grated nutmeg
- 1.5 liters vegetable stock
- 450g spinach, washed, roots removed
- 150g kale leaves, washed
- 1 head of broccoli, sliced
- 1 lemon, juice of 1 lemon

Serve with, crispy tofu pieces, toasted nuts, and seeds, fried onion, and toasted ciabatta slices

DIRECTIONS

1. Heat the olive oil in a large saucepan or soup pot over medium heat. Add the onion, garlic, celery, and carrot. Cook for 5 minutes until tender. Stir in the rice and add the cumin, mixed spice, and nutmeg. Stir-fry for 1-2 minutes.
2. Add half of the stock and simmer for 8 minutes. Press the drained spinach, kale, and broccoli into the saucepan, cover and when the leaves have wilted pour in the rest of the stock. Bring up to a boil, turn it down immediately, and simmer for 10 minutes.
3. Puree in a high-speed blender or food processor. Add back to the cleaned saucepan and stir in the lemon juice, and season to taste with freshly ground black pepper and salt. Keep warm while preparing toppings. Before serving stir in cream or yogurt if preferred.
4. Serve crispy tofu pieces, toasted nuts and seeds, fried onion and toasted ciabatta slices.

Brewing Greenlandic hot coffee in a Bordeaux glass is a good option to get by during winter.

NEW HAMPSHIRE, USA

New Hampshireis a unique state in the United States with a current population of 1,405,243 people.

An abundance of maple syrup, scenic deserts, and serene towns are typical of the mountain state.

White Mountain Forest, the glory of the sports in winter season is a favorite hang-out spot for lovers of adventure.

Its state capital is called Concord.

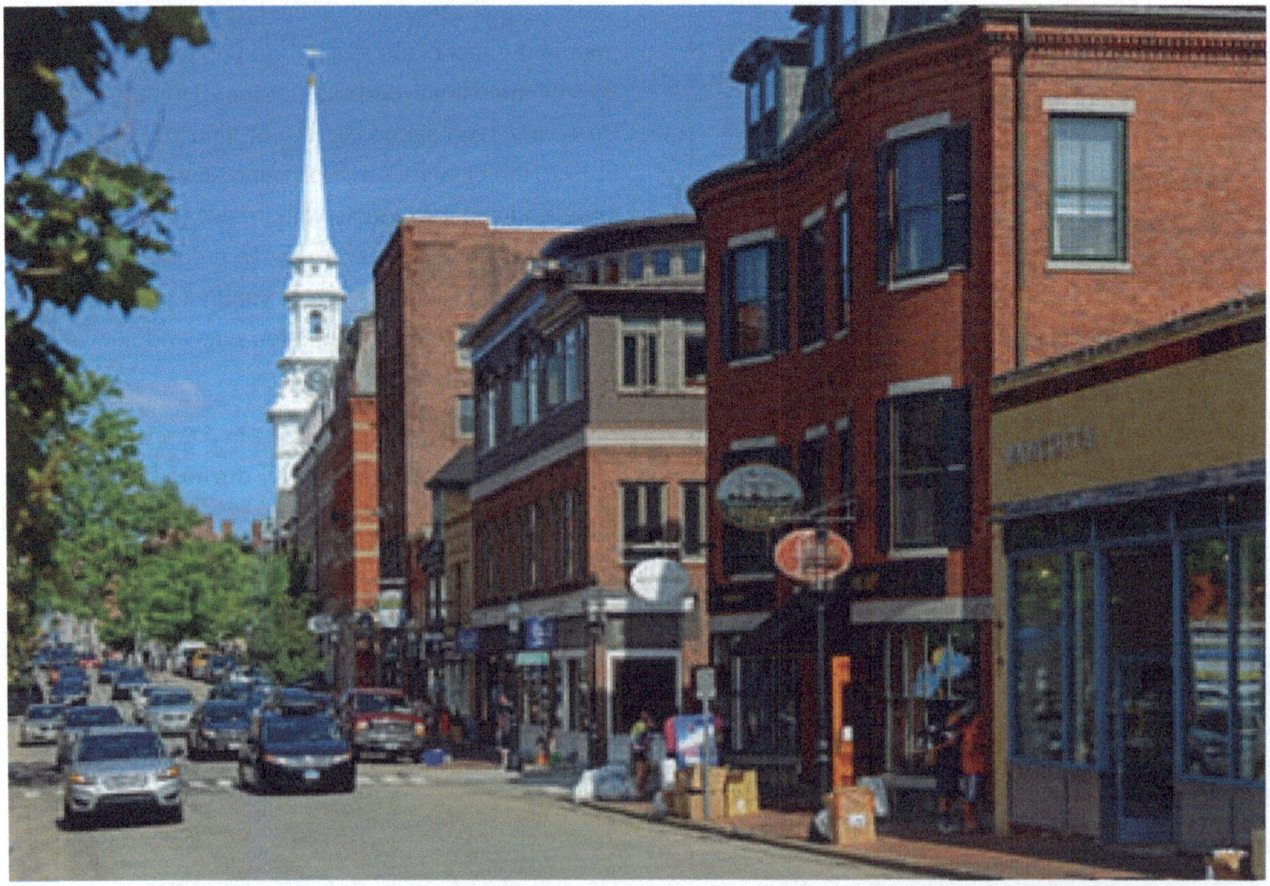

Irish Beef Stew

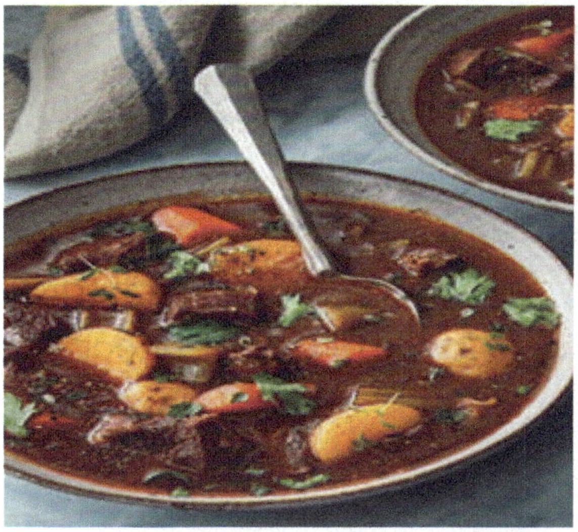

Amount of calories per serving of Irish beef stew is 235.

Sometimes even the best winter soups can be lacking in the kind of hearty heft we need to get us through the winter.
This Irish Beef Stew goes from ordinary to outstanding with the addition of a cup of Guinness stout. Adding root vegetables like turnips or parsnips will make it extra hearty.

INGREDIENTS

- 2 pounds lean beef stew or chuck, in 2-inch chunks
- 1 teaspoon salt
- 1/2 teaspoon pepper
- flour for dredging
- 2 tablespoons bacon drippings or vegetable oil
- 2 large yellow onions, chopped
- 1 garlic clove, finely minced (optional)
- 6 to 8 medium carrots, scraped and sliced
- 2 to 3 large potatoes, peeled and cut into cubes
- 2 to 3 turnips, peeled and cut into cubes (optional)
- 1 cup Guinness stout
- 1 cup beef broth

DIRECTIONS

1. Season beef with salt and pepper; toss beef chunks in flour until well coated.
2. Heat drippings or oil in a Dutch oven and brown beef over medium-high heat in two batches. When all are browned, remove beef from the pan and add onions and garlic.
3. Cook over medium heat until onions are translucent.
4. Return beef to pot and add carrots, potatoes, turnips, stout, and broth. Bring to a boil and reduce heat to a simmer. Cover and cook for 2 hours or until beef is tender.

A stroll to North Hampshire's Mount Washington will give you the windiest experience of your lifetime

OAXACA, MEXICO

Oaxaca also called the city of Oaxaca de Juárez with a population of 726,000. The weather here is pretty inviting and tourist-friendly. The scenic waterfalls of Hierve el Agua are said to connect to warm water bodies.

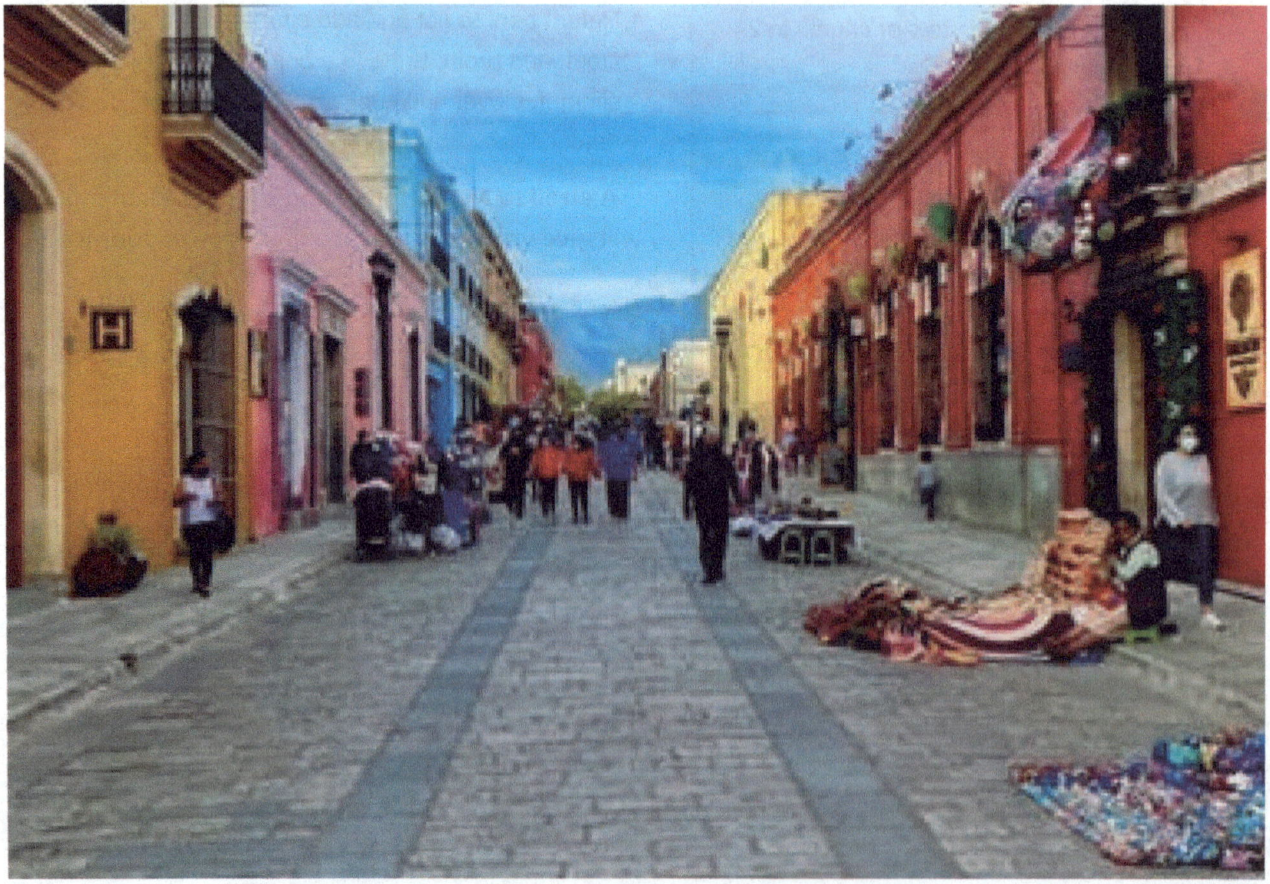

Mexican Noodle Soup (Sopa de Fideo)

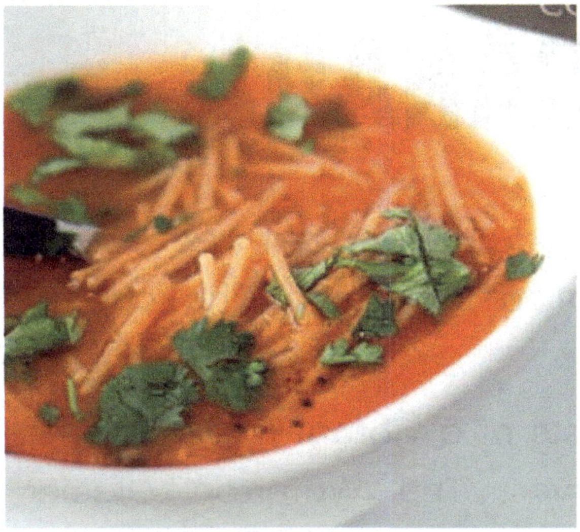

The ultimate comfort food, and every Mexican child's favorite soup.
Short angel-hair noodles are fried until golden brown, then simmered in an onion, garlic, and tomato puree.
Once the noodles begin absorbing the puree, vegetable stock is added, and everything is simmered until the noodles are tender.
You can add zucchini or your vegetable of choice. Serve with wedges of lime. It is a warm comforting soup made with a tangy tomato base and golden brown noodles. Kids love it!

INGREDIENTS

- 1 tbsp. Oil (optional)
- 8 oz. Angel hair pasta or whole wheat thin spaghetti, broken into 1 in. pieces
- 1 can (14.5 oz) Diced tomatoes or 2 cups of fresh diced tomatoes
- ½ Onion, white, chopped
- 3 Garlic cloves, peeled
- 10 cups Vegetable stock
- 1 Mexican zucchini, diced
- 1 Lime, cut into quarters

DIRECTIONS

1. In a medium pot get your vegetable stock boiling hot and set aside.
2. Set a large pot to medium heat and add oil. Once the oil is hot add broken-up noodles and toss to coat in oil. Continue to cook until noodles are golden brown, about 3 minutes.
3. While the noodles are browning, place the tomatoes, onion, garlic, and 2 cups of vegetable stock in the blender and process until smooth.
4. Strain this mixture directly into the golden noodles still in the hot pot. Stir to prevent the noodles from sticking.
5. Let the mixture simmer for 1 minute. Add the rest of your stock and set heat to high. Add zucchini and cook noodles at a low boil until noodles are al dente and zucchini is tender. Stir often. Season.
6. Serve with a wedge of lime so everyone can add as much lime juice as they like.

The choicest of places to visit during winter while sipping a glass of Oaxacan hot toddy.

ALBERTA, CANADA

Thinking of a Province to visit in Canada? You might just wish to visit Alberta. The capital city is called Edmonton. The current population is estimated at 4.46 million.

This Western Canada province boasts of a vibrant forest, serene lakes, and wealthy mineral reserves. The Waterton Glacier International Peace screams biodiversity to an average tourist.

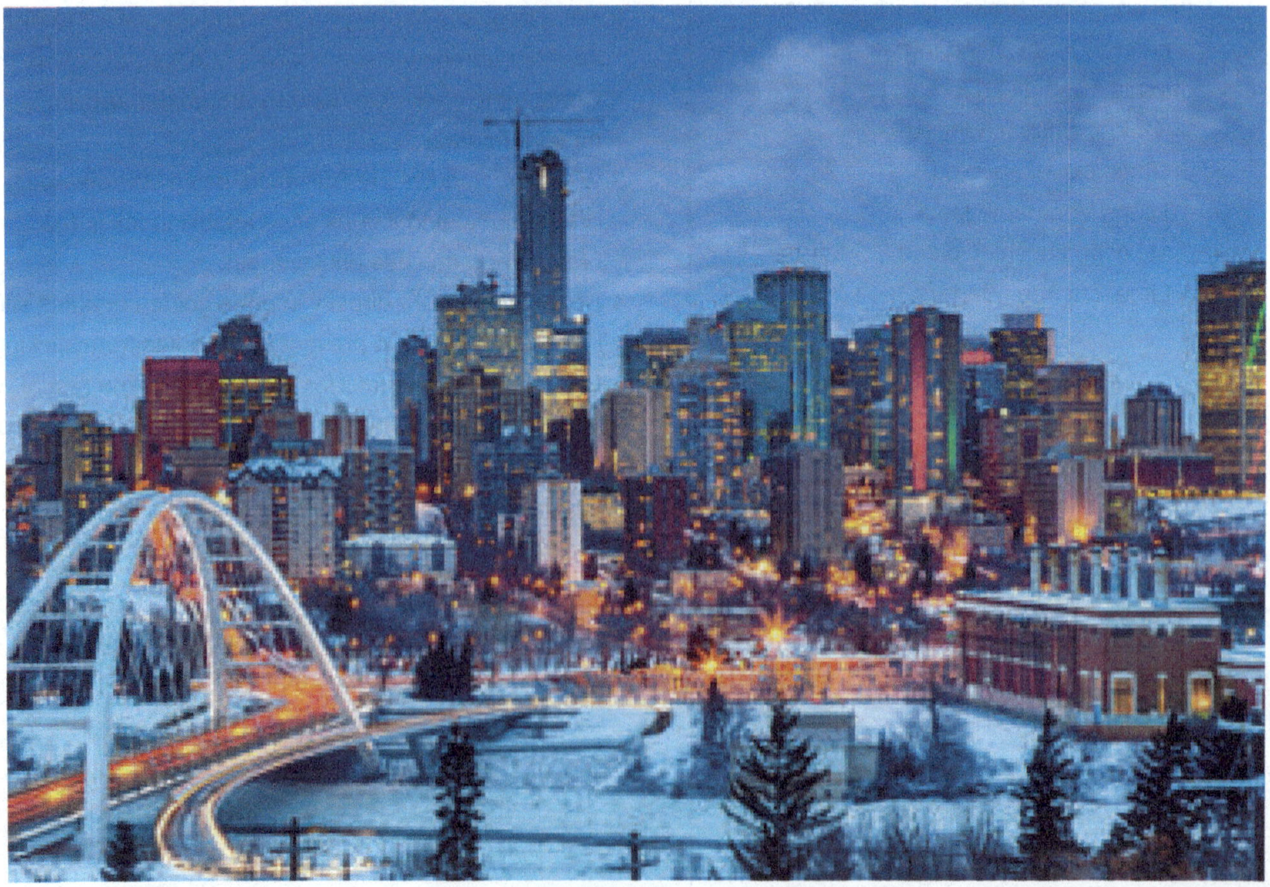

Easy Chicken Curry Soup

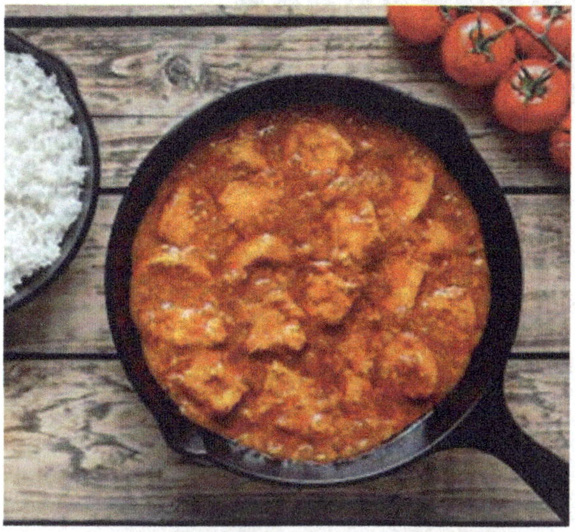

Amount of calories per serving of Mexican Noodle Soup is 352.

INGREDIENTS

- 1 tbsp(15 ml) vegetable oil
- ¼ cup (60 ml) water
- 2 medium onions, chopped
- 6 cloves garlic, crushed or finely
- chopped
- 1 tbsp (15 ml) curry powder
- 2 tbsp (30 ml) garam masala
- ½ tsp (2 ml) salt (optional)
- 19 oz (540 ml) can of tomatoes
- (whole or chopped)
- ¼ cup (60 ml) packed fresh cilantro,
- finely chopped
- 1 cup (250 ml) unflavored low-fat yogurt
- 1 cup (250 ml) of chicken stock (1
- package reduced salt bouillon + 1
- cup/250 ml water)
- 18 skinned chicken drumsticks or
- thighs, skin removed (3½ lbs/1.7 kg
- weight with skin and bones or
- 3 lbs/1.5 kg weight with skin removed)
- ¼ cup (60 ml) fresh cilantro,
- roughly chopped, for topping

Chili loves pumpkin and chocolate! Use these fun ingredients to help revitalize an old favorite. The pumpkin adds fiber and body while the chocolate and cocoa powder blend in creating a rich, smooth soup.

DIRECTIONS

1. To a large heavy pot, heat the oil and water at low to medium. Add the
2. onions and garlic to the pot. Cook until soft. Add the spices, stirring
3. frequently, and cook for one or two minutes until the spices are well blended. Add a bit of water if too dry.
4. Add to the pot, the tomatoes, cilantro, yogurt, and chicken stock. Blend
5. together, then add the chicken pieces.
6. Cover the pot and simmer gently at low-medium heat. Stir periodically. Cook
7. for 1–1½ hour, or until chicken is cooked. If too thick, add extra chicken
8. stock or water if needed. If too thin, cook for the last 15–30 minutes
9. without the lid.
10. After cooking, add chopped cilantro

Your trip to Alberta is incomplete without touring Banff National Park!
Undoubtedly, a stop-over at Athabasca falls will leave you with a lifetime experience.

SPRING SOUPS

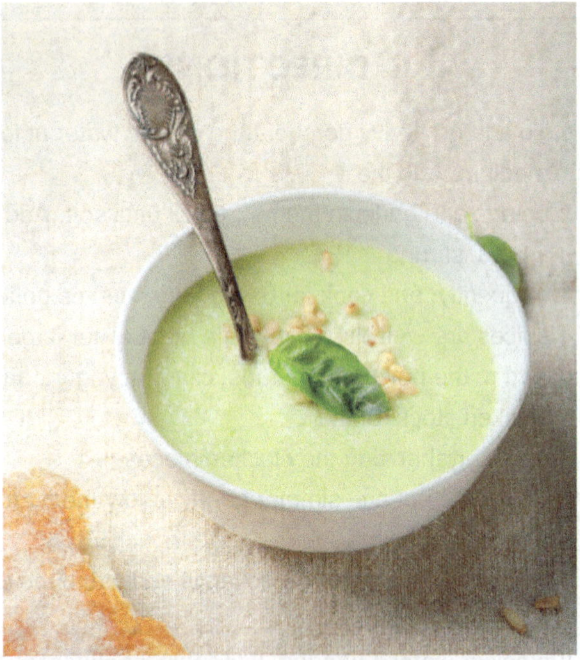
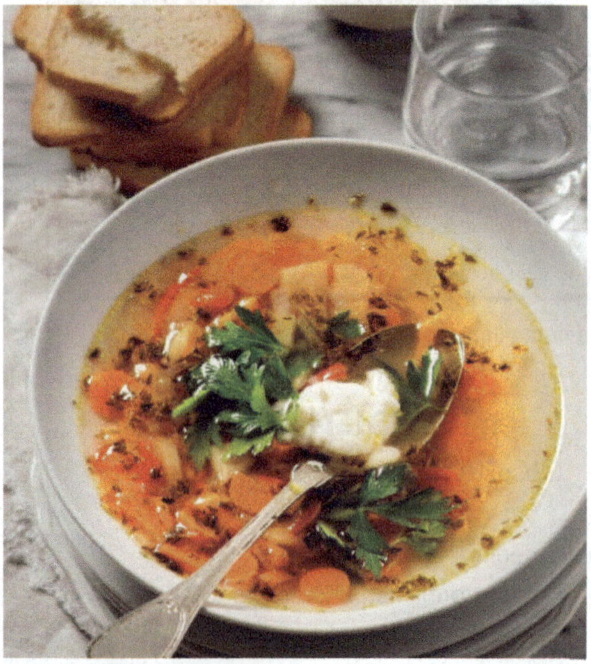
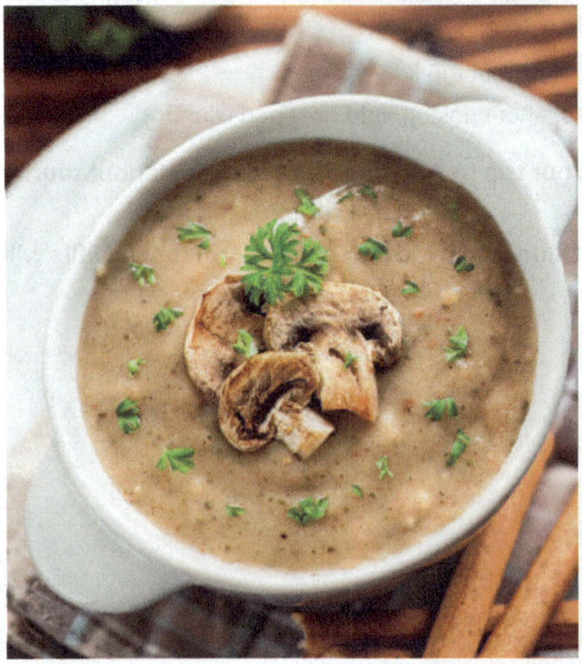
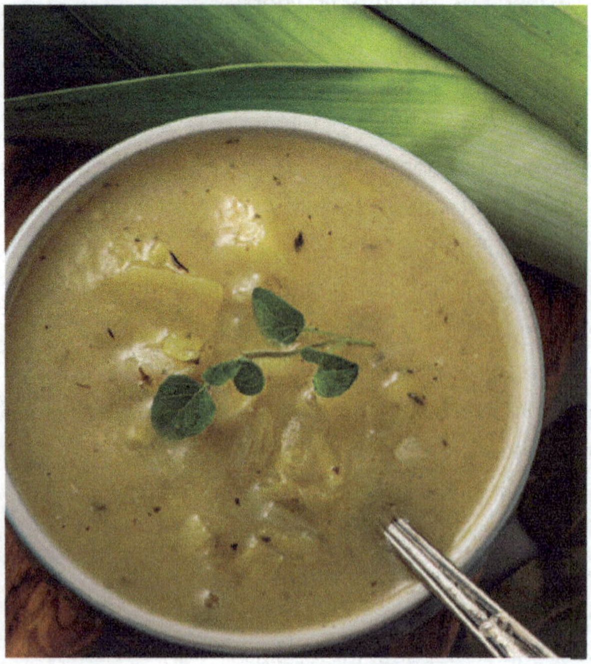

GREENLAND

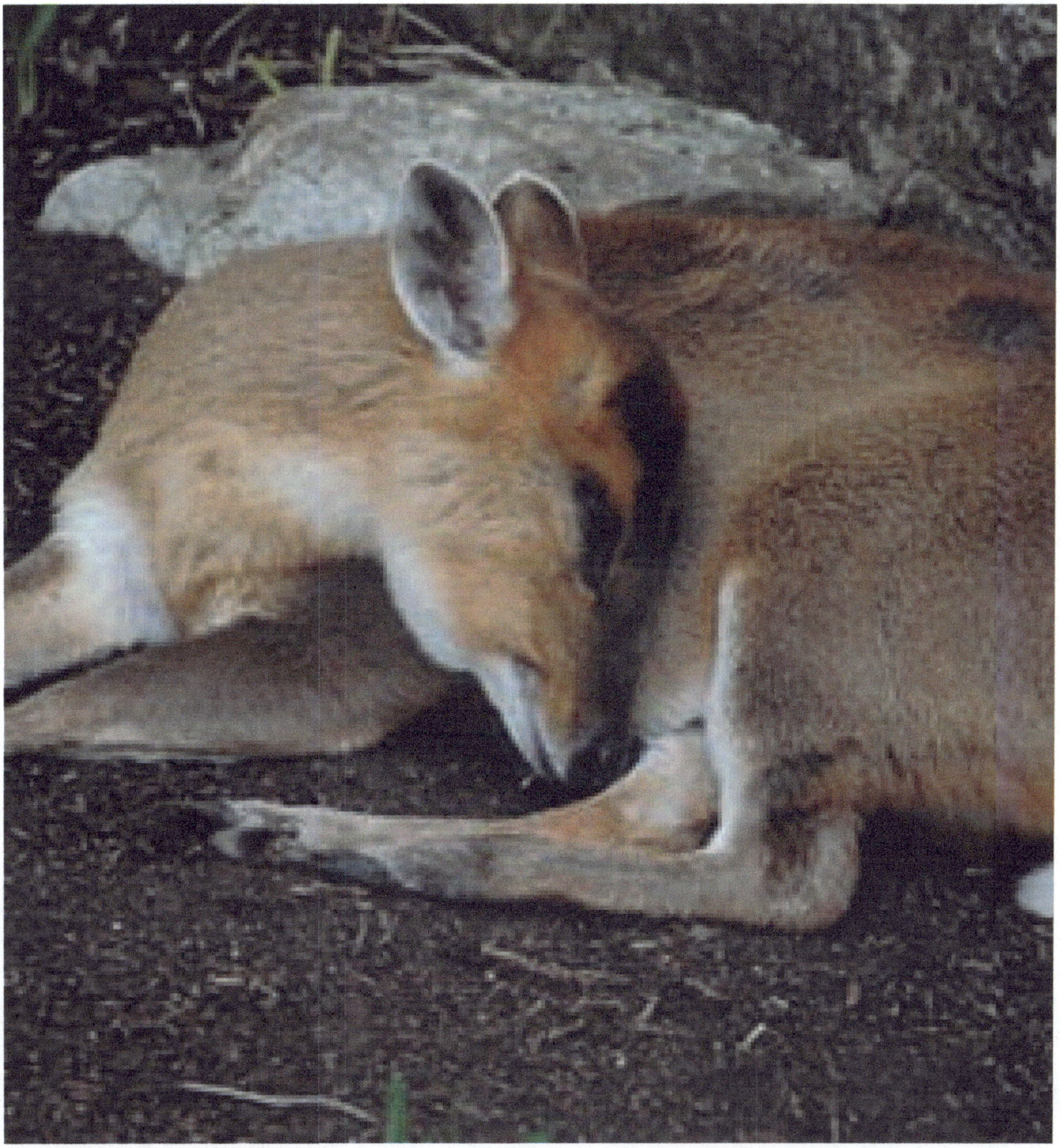

Fish Soup for Spring

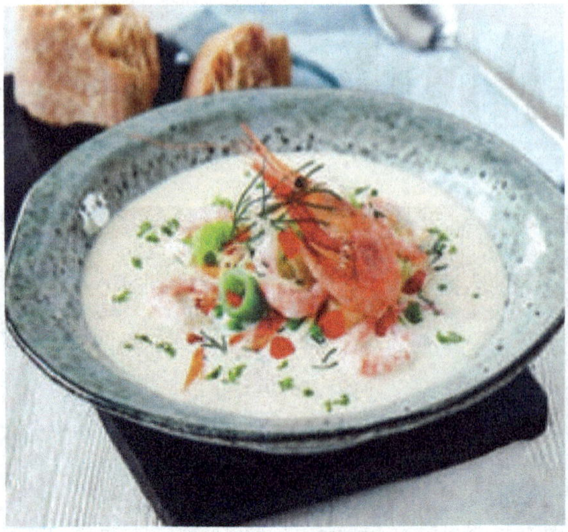

Each serving contains 152 Calories.

INGREDIENTS

- 1200 ml of fish stock
- 600 ml of dry white wine
- 4 shallots, finely chopped
- 600 ml cream
- 2100 g shell-on prawns
- 2 bulbs of fennel
- 1 bunch of finely chopped spring onions
- 6 carrots, peeled
- 225 g peas
- 6 tomatoes
- 1 bunch of finely chopped chervil

Greenland's fish soup with shell-on prawns and crunchy vegetable prawns.
Embrace the beauty of spring with a creamy bowl of fish soup packed with fineness, flavor, and colorful aquatic dainties like this.

DIRECTIONS

1. Boil together the white wine and finely chopped shallots until there is about half the liquid remaining. Add the fish stock and cook for a further 5 minutes or so. Add the cream and cook until approx. 2 liters remain. Season with salt and pepper to taste.
2. Peel the shell-on prawns. If you wish, save 10-20 prawns for garnishing. Chop the carrots, spring onions, and fennel into small pieces. Seed the tomatoes and finely dice them. Add the vegetables and prawns to the soup and bring to a boil. Add chervil and peas and season with salt and pepper.
3. Serve with bread.

Sipping ice beer will not be a bad idea to embrace all the goodness of Greenland!

COLORADO, USA

Also known as the Centennial State a populationof 5.85 million people. Its largest city, Denver is also its capital and center of finance.

Dry wilderness plains, snow-top mountains, and bustling towns are typical of this western U. Sstate. Springtime is a great time to sample the serenity of the Colorado Springs

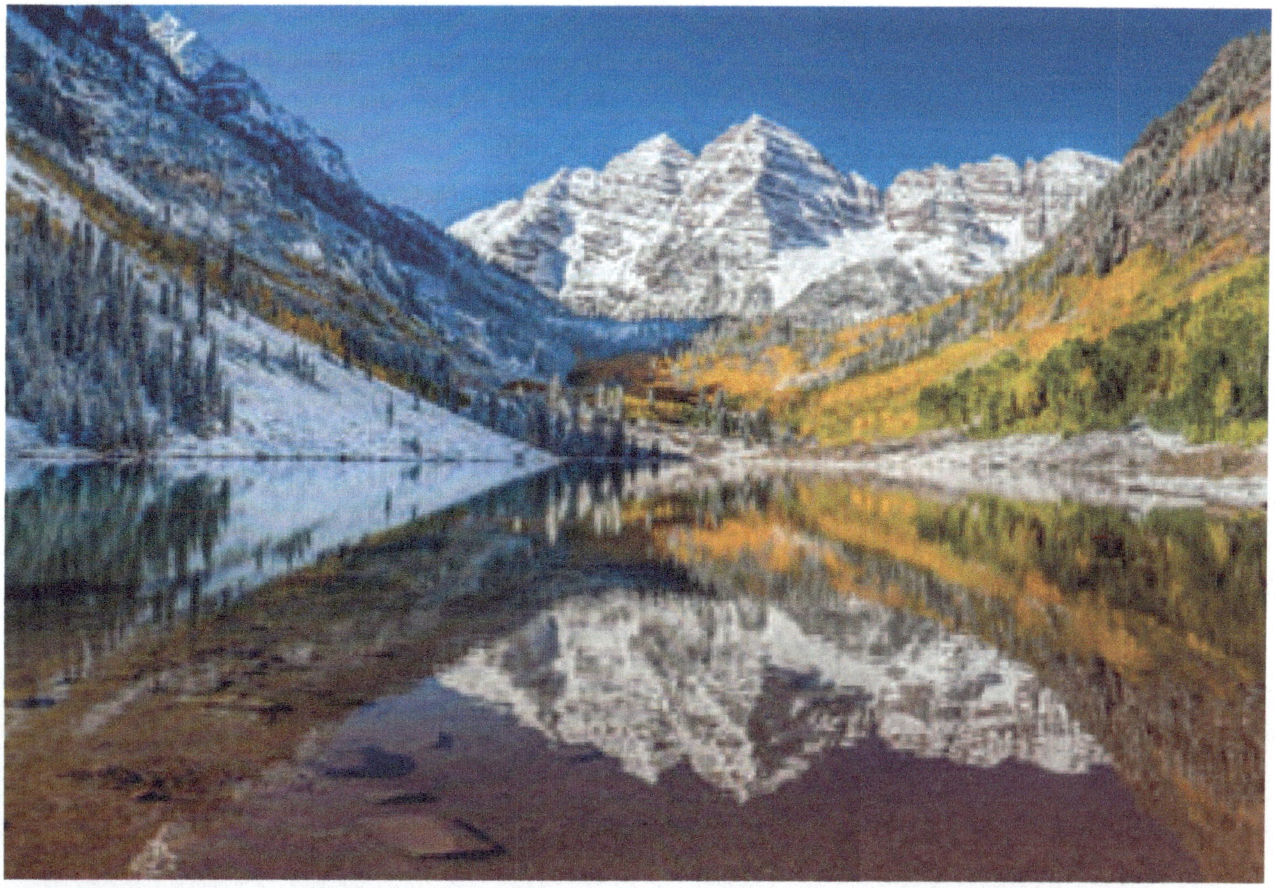

Sweet Potato, Chickpea & Kale Coconut Curry Soup

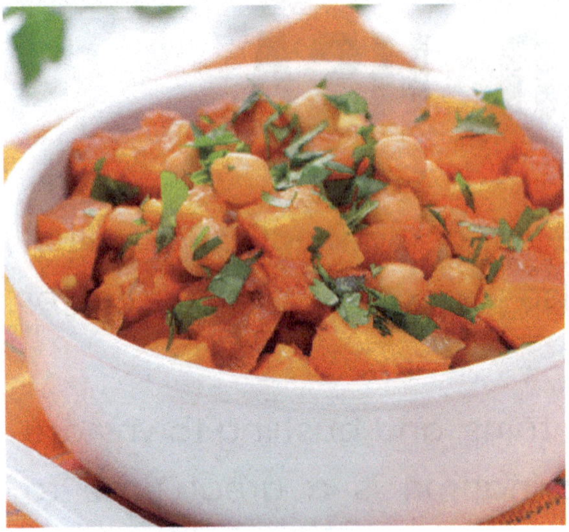

INGREDIENTS

- 3 sweet potatoes
- 1 small yellow onion, diced
- 1 large carrot, diced
- 1-inch nub of fresh ginger minced
- 3 garlic cloves, crushed
- 1 tablespoon curry powder
- 1 teaspoon ground cumin
- 1 teaspoon garam masala
- 1/4 teaspoon ground ginger
- 1/4 tsp ground turmeric
- 1 (15-ounce) can of coconut milk
- 2 (15-ounce) cans of vegetable stock
- 1 1/2 cups cooked chickpeas
- 1 1/2 cups finely chopped kale
- 1 lime
- 1/4 cup chopped cilantro
- Salt, pepper, cooking oil
- Honey or sugar to taste (optional)

This hearty soup is brewing a lot of sweetness for your springtime fantasies.

DIRECTIONS

1. Heat a few tablespoons of cooking oil in a large heavy-bottom pan on medium heat. Add onion and carrot and cook for a few minutes until soft and translucent then add the ginger and crushed garlic. Cook for another minute.
2. Add all the spices and cook for 20 seconds, stirring, until fragrant. Add the sweet potato, coconut milk, and vegetable stock. Bring to a simmer and leave for about 20-25 minutes until the sweet potato is soft.
3. When the sweet potato is soft (pierce with a knife to check) blend the soup with a hand-held blender until slightly smooth, leaving some texture. Add the drained chickpeas and kale and cook at a low simmer for 10-15 minutes more. Add the cilantro and, juice from the lime, and add salt and pepper to taste. Add sweetener if needed.

A chilled glass of a fifty-niner drink in one of Colorado's warmest springs will soothe your tensed nerves.

It might interest you to know that this region plays home to the world's largest natural hot springs!

PUEBLA

This city is in the southeast of Mexico City.

Delicious cuisine, pre-historic pottery, and medieval architecture are just a part of this city with an estimated population of about 3,295,000.

You may wish to stop over at Fonda de Santa Clara's to satisfy your local cravings.

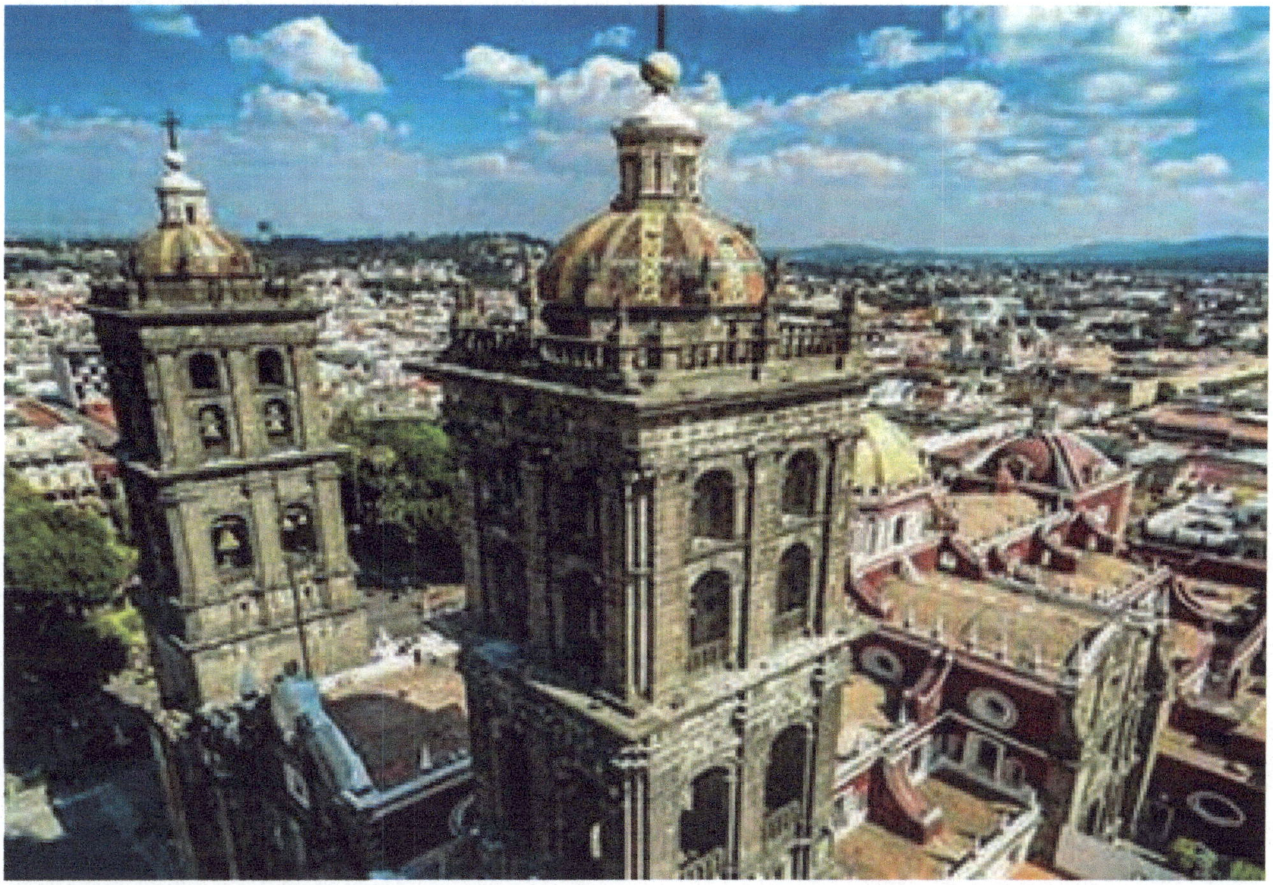

Vegetable Soup with Radish Sauce

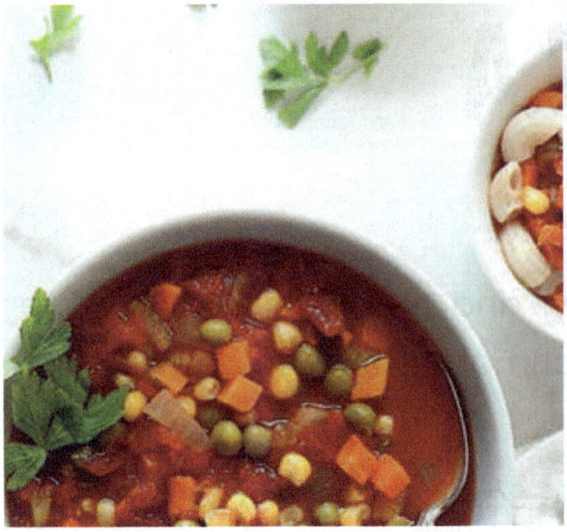

Amount of calories in vegetable soup with radish sauce is 99.9 calories.

INGREDIENTS

- 1 1/2 lbs. (750 g) boneless pork shoulder, cubed
- 1/2 white onion
- 3 cloves garlic
- 10 cups (80 floz/2.5 l) water
- 2 tablespoons sea salt
- 1 1/2 lbs. (750 g) tomatillos, husks removed
- 1 cup (1 1/2 oz/45 g) chopped fresh cilantro
- 3 ears corn, each cut into 3 chunks
- 8 ozs. (250 g) small zucchini, sliced 1/2 inch (1 cm) thick
- 8 ozs. (250 g) young green beans, trimmed and cut in half
- For the sauce
- 1 cup (8fl. oz/250 ml) water
- 1 tablespoon sea salt
- 1 tablespoon vinegar
- 4 chilespoblanos, roasted, peeled, membranes removed, and cut into thin strips
- 6 radishes, finely chopped
- 1/2 cup (4 oz/125 g) finely chopped white onion
- 3/4 cup (6 floz/180 ml) freshly squeezed orange juice
- 1/2 cup (4 floz/125 ml) freshly squeezed lime juice

There are no specific foods or dishes associated with Cinco de Mayo, but since it is springtime, here is a vegetable soup from Puebla made special by the addition of a zesty radish sauce.

This dish is a complete and flavorful meal traditionally cooked in a clay pot.

DIRECTIONS

1. Place the pork, onion, garlic, water, and salt in a large pot or Dutch oven. Bring to a boil, skim the surface, reduce the heat, and simmer, covered, until the pork is tender, about 45 minutes. Correct the seasonings and set aside.
2. In a blender, puree the tomatillos, cilantro, and chilesserranos. Set aside.
3. To make the sauce, combine the water, salt and vinegar in a bowl, add the chilespoblanos and soak for 30 minutes. Drain the chiles and combine with the radishes, onion, orange juice,and lime juice.
4. Twenty minutes before serving, bring the pork mixture to a boil, add the corn, zucchini, and green beans and simmer until the vegetables are tender, 10-15 minutes. Bring the soup to a boil, add the tomatillo puree, stir and remove from the heat.
5. Pass the sauce separately, to be served over the hot soup.

Bebida de puebla is a liquor you must not miss on your next visit to Puebla.

Lovers of pottery will be interested to know that Puebla is the first place in the world where Talavera ceramics was found.

BRITISH COLUMBIA, CANADA

This is Canada's westernmost province, with a current population of about 4.7 million people.

This province is defined by its unique mountains, defined pacific coastlines. Its capital town is called Victoria.

Hikers will love it at the Glaciers National Park. The buoyant economy of this province thrives on mining, forestry, and film production.

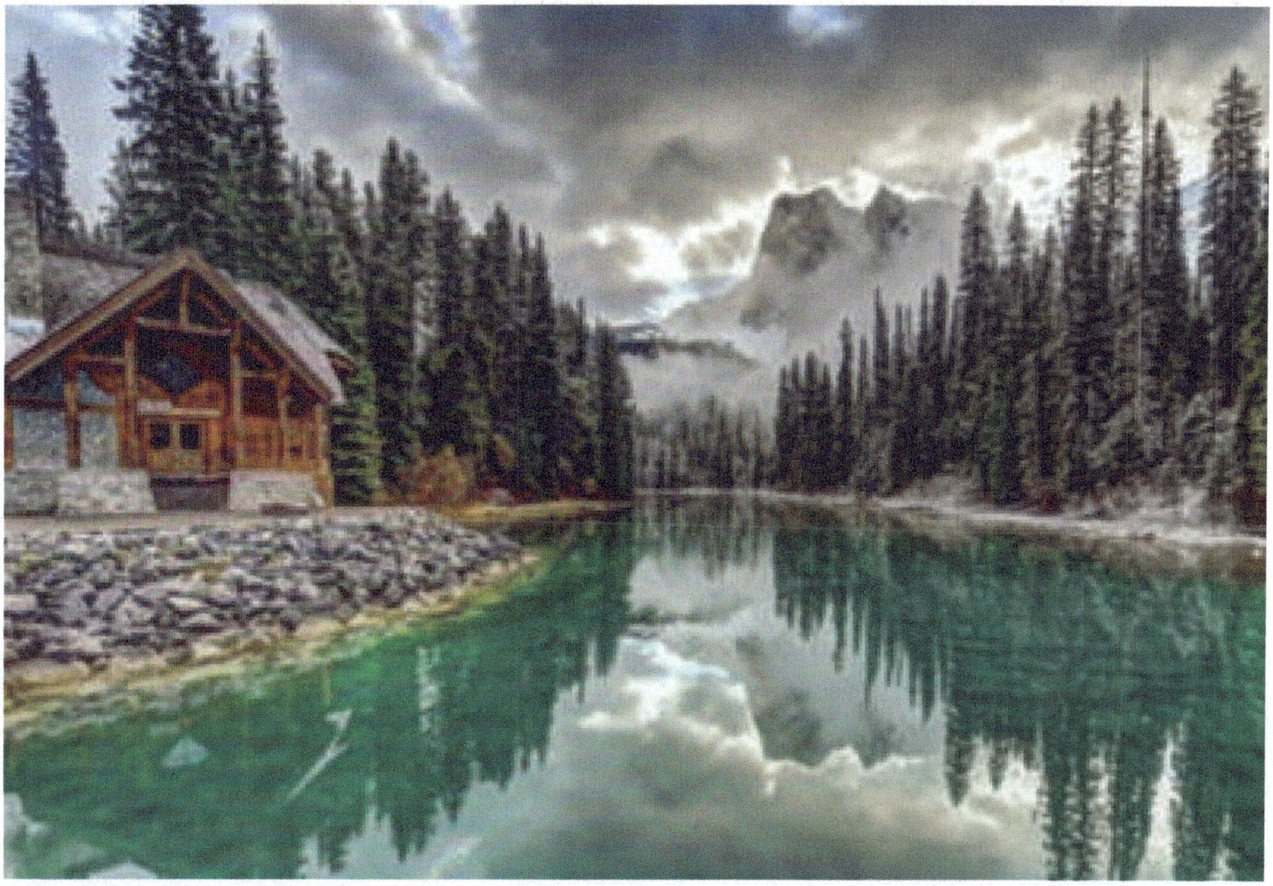

Simple Lemony Chicken Soup with Spring Veggies

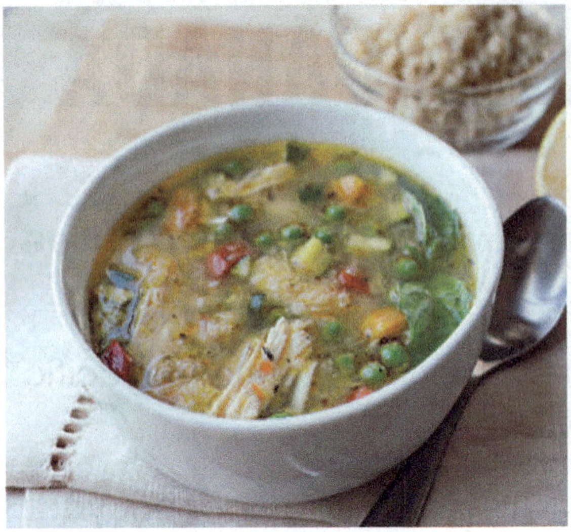

This chicken soup with spring veggies and a delightful hint of lemon is a light and healthy meal, simply prepared in under forty minutes and brimming with lots of bright flavors!
In that in-between time when the cold weather begins to move out and make way for warmer days.
This chicken soup is so comforting, enlivening the palate with a hint of brightness and the flavor of the fresh produce that is on hand and plentiful.

INGREDIENTS

- 2 tablespoons butter
- 1 tablespoon olive oil
- 1 leek, quartered, and white part sliced
- 2 carrots, peeled and diced small (if you can find multi-colored carrots, those are beautiful)
- 2 cloves garlic, pressed through garlic press
- Salt
- Black pepper
- 1 teaspoon Herbes de Provence
- 4 cups warm chicken stock/broth
- 1 cup fresh English peas (or frozen peas)
- 1 cup baby zucchini, small dice
- 2 cups cooked chicken, shredded or cubed
- 2 teaspoons lemon zest
- 2 tablespoons fresh lemon juice
- 2 cups cooked quinoa
- ¼ cup chopped, fresh basil leaves
- 4 lemon wedges, garnish

DIRECTIONS

1. Place a medium-large soup pot over medium heat, and add in the butter and olive oil; once melted, add in the sliced leek and diced carrots, and sweat for about 3-5 minutes, or until slightly tender and the leeks are becoming translucent.
2. Add in the garlic, and once that becomes aromatic, add in a pinch or two of salt and pepper, and the herbs de Provence; stir to combine.
3. Next, add in the warm chicken stock or broth, and bring to a gentle simmer; cover partially with a lid, and cook for about 15-20 minutes, or until carrots are tender.
4. Turn the heat off; add in the English peas (or frozen peas), the diced baby zucchini, the shredded or cubed chicken, and the lemon zest and juice; stir to combine, and allow the peas/zucchini to become crisp-tender and bright green in the hot stock, about 3-4 minutes; check to see if additional salt or pepper is needed.
5. To serve, add about ½ cup of the cooked quinoa to a bowl, and ladle some of the soup with the veggies and chicken over top; sprinkle over some of the fresh basil, and squeeze in some additional lemon juice from the lemon wedge garnish, if desired.

Find yourself quickly to the Pacific Rim National Park Reserve for an experience of British Colombia.

Stanley Park or Vancouver Islands are exciting choices too!

SUMMER SOUPS

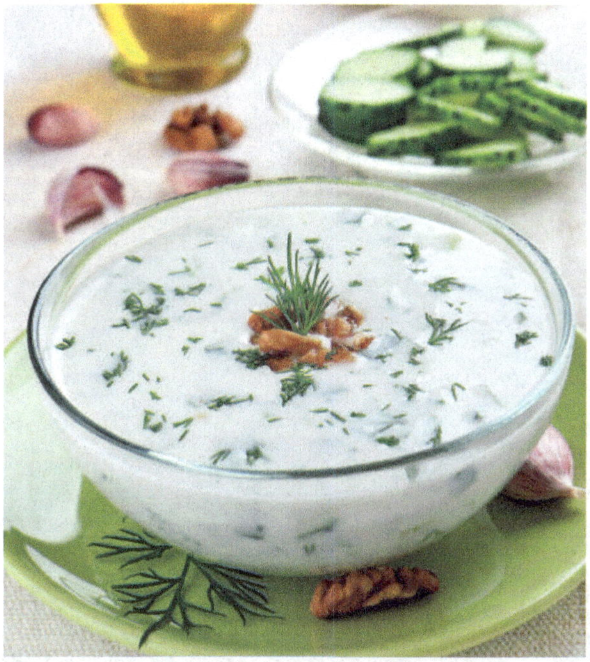
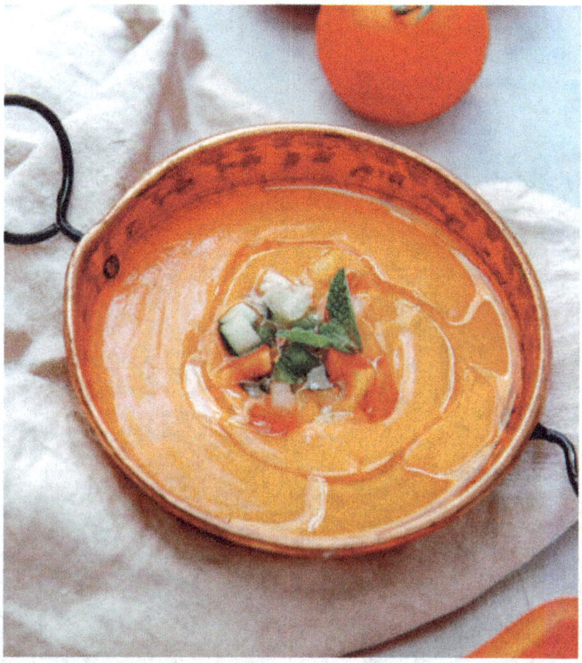
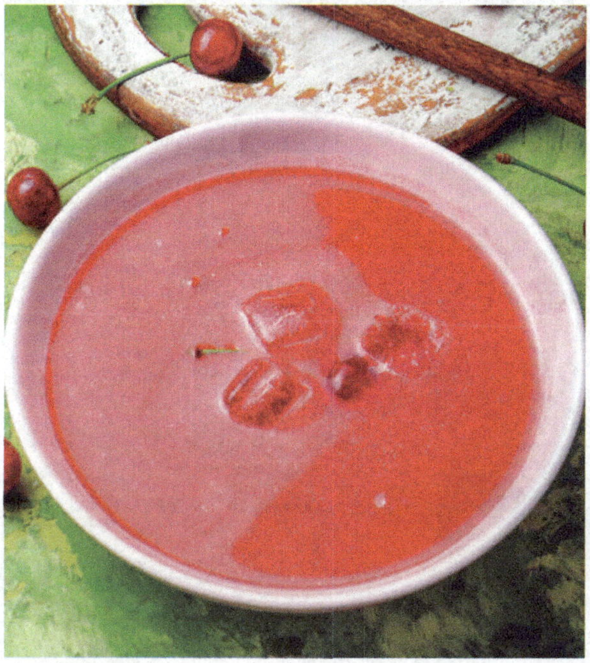
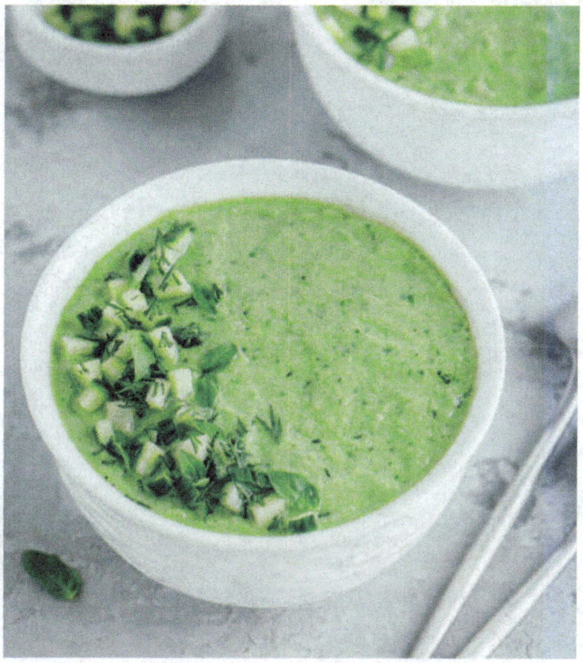

GREENLAND

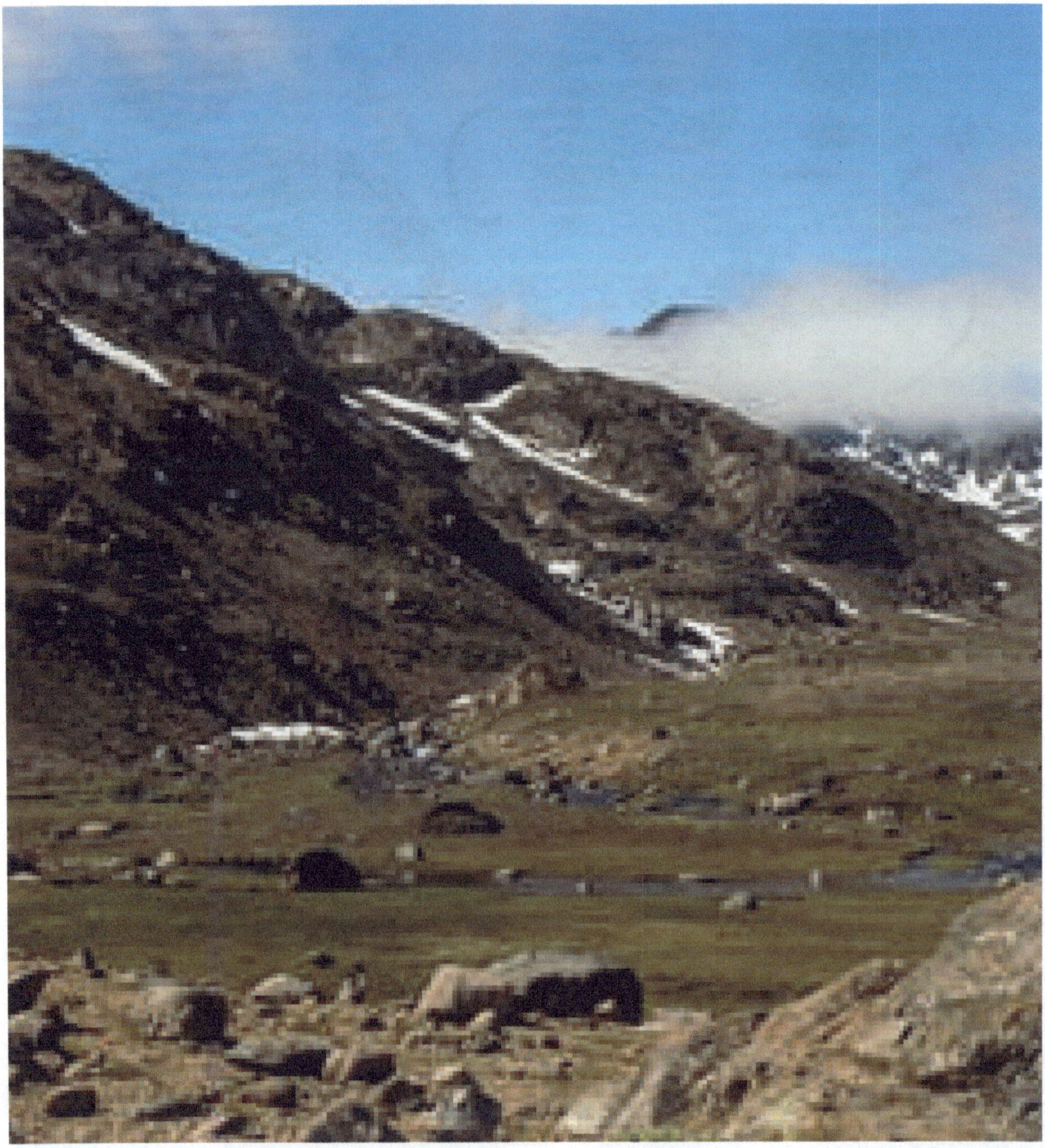

Lamb Soup for Summer

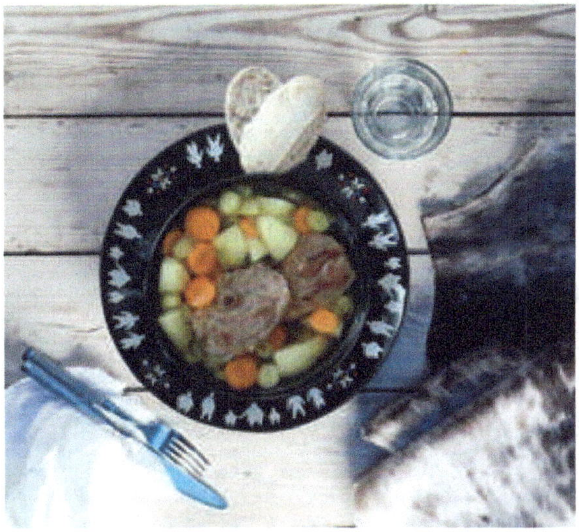

Amount of calories per serving is 262 calories.

INGREDIENTS

- ½ kg of lamb
- 1 onion
- 4 carrots
- ½ stalk of celery
- 4 medium-sized potatoes
- 3 smaller turnips
- 1 large leek – or a bag of frozen soup herbs
- Butter/margarine and olive oil
- Salt and pepper

The avalanche of roaming lambs on the pastures feeding on the greenish meadows during summer may have inspired this tasty lamb soup recipe. It is always an awesome summer delight for Greenlanders.

DIRECTIONS

1. Cut all the vegetables to the desired size.
2. The butter is browned, and oil is added to the pan.
3. Brown the lamb on both sides. When the meat has been browned, remove it from the pan.
4. Cook the vegetables in the pan.
5. Add the meat back to the vegetables and add 1 liter of water or until the water covers the contents of the pot. Simmer for an hour.
6. The dish is served with coarse bread / flütes.

The Greenland excitement is incomplete without loving the wonders of the Glacier monument in Northeast Greenland National Park.

It plays home to polar bears, bearded seals and arctic hares.

LOS ANGELES, USA

The bustling city and home to most of the United States cinematography is in South California.

With a population of over 4 million people, the 2nd largest city in the United States is a major social hub in American culture.

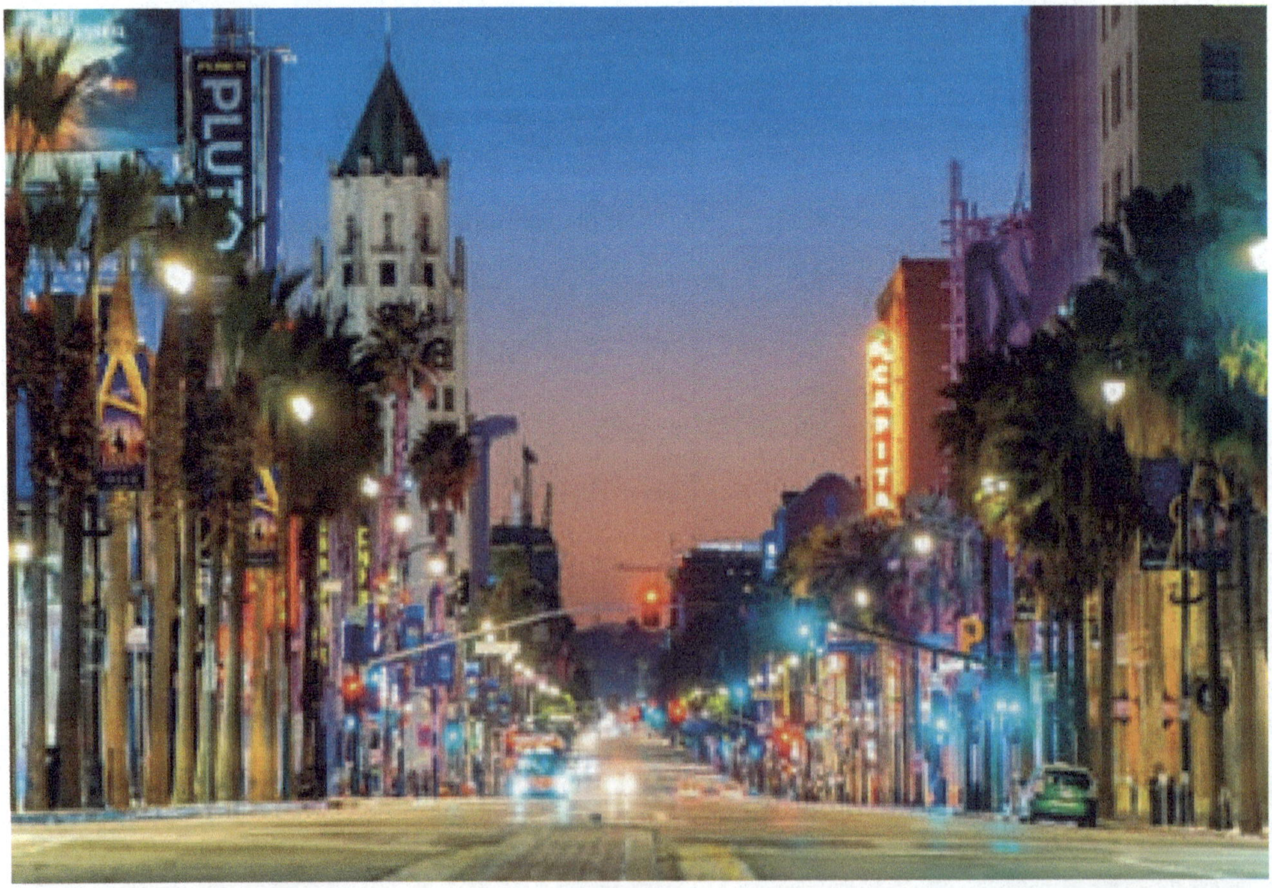

Chilled Cucumber Soup

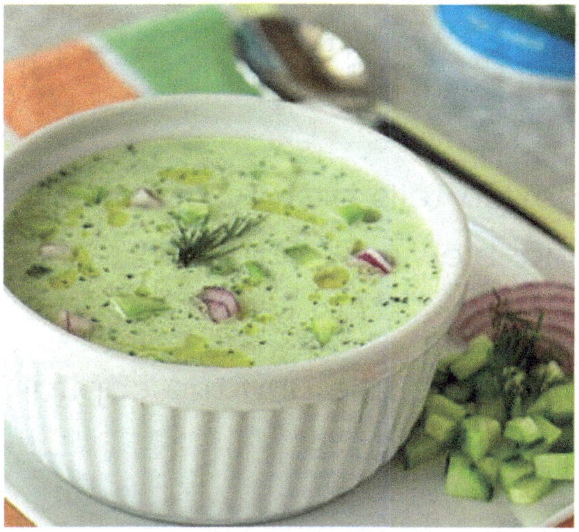

Amount of calories per serving is 96.

INGREDIENTS

- 2 large cucumbers
- 2 tbsp chopped onion
- 1/2 cup buttermilk
- 1/4 cup sour cream
- 1 tablespoon rice vinegar
- 1 tablespoon extra virgin olive oil
- 2 tablespoons fresh dill, chopped
- 1/2 teaspoon kosher salt
- Pinch black pepper

Good news for calories-conscious folks. This 10-minute zero-heat yumminess is super easy to prepare plus it's very tasty.
Cold and refreshing, cucumber soup is a great recipe for a hot summer day.

DIRECTIONS

1. Prep the cucumbers, onion, and dill:
2. Peel, seed, and roughly chop the cucumbers. Chop the onion and dill. Blend:
3. Put all the ingredients into a blender and pulse until completely smooth. Adjust seasonings to taste. Add more salt and pepper if needed.
4. At this point you can make ahead and chill in a container in the refrigerator until cold.
5. Pour into bowls and garnish with a drizzle of olive oil and dill.

Perhaps sipping your favorite brand of wine at the Tropicana pool will release that soothing effect to your tensed muscles.

Los Angeles will sure keep you active from the first day.

CHIAPAS, MEXICO

The mountainous state in southern Mexico tells a story of historic archaeology, scenic forestry, mind-blowing artifacts, and everything social diversity.

With a current population of over 6 million people and the capital city as Tuxtla Gutiérrez, Chiapas boasts of highlands.

Desirous to view ancient ruins?

Come over to Chiapas to marvel at the crashing Maya ruins of long ago!

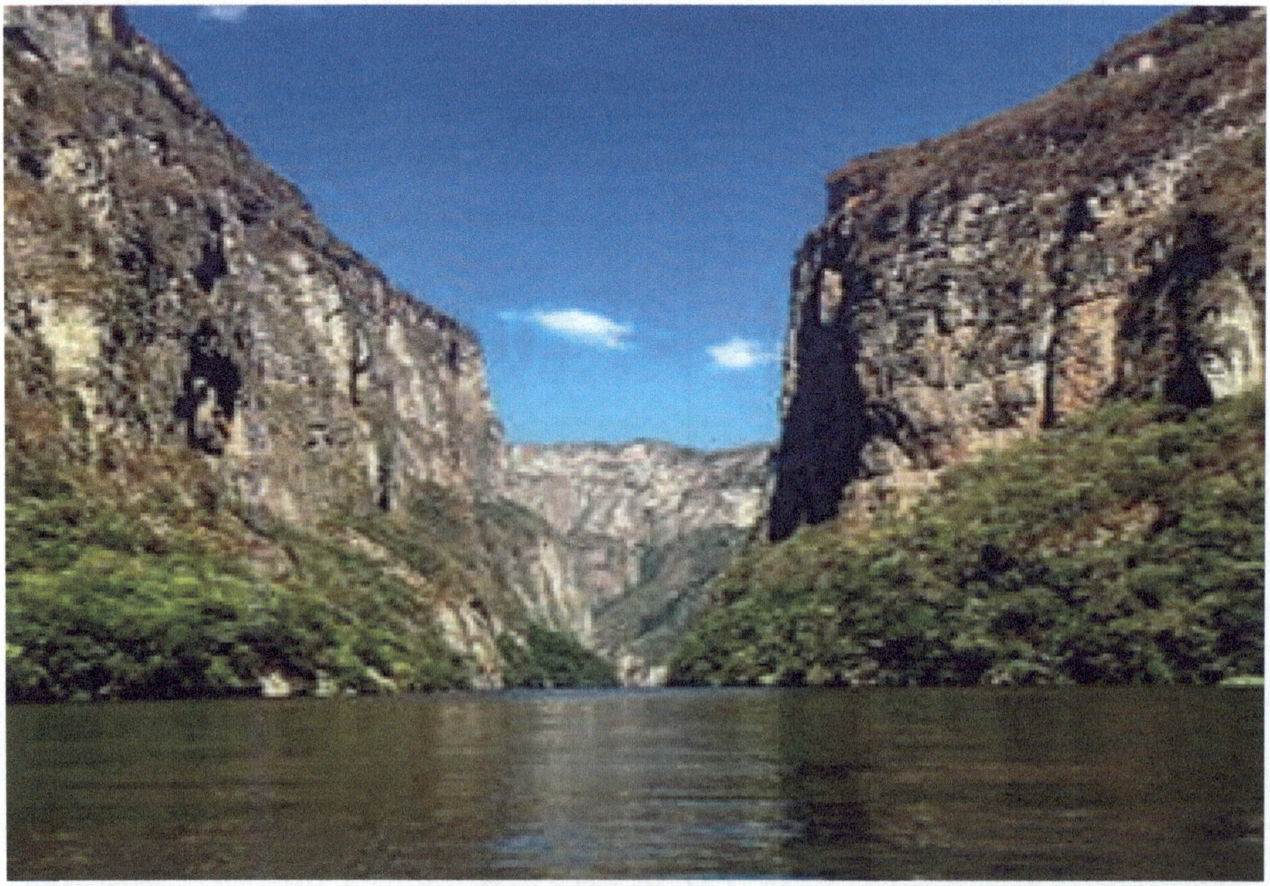

Corn and Zucchini Soup

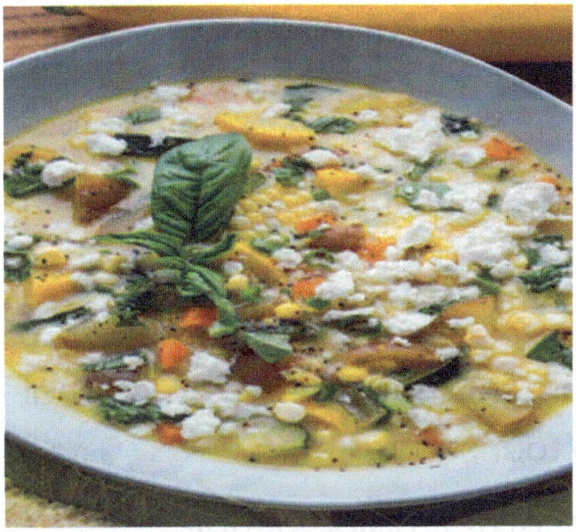

Amount of calories per serving is 100.

INGREDIENTS

- 2 medium zucchinis, chopped
- 4 cups vegetable or chicken stock
- 310g can creamed corn
- ½ cup low-fat evaporated milk

Not to be corny, but this light soup is delicious.

Use fresh, frozen, or canned corn – whatever fits the season and your budget.

DIRECTIONS

1. Place zucchini and stock in a large pot and bring to a boil.
2. Simmer over a gentle heat for 10 minutes or until zucchini is tender.
3. Remove from heat, puree in a blender until smooth.
4. Stir through creamed corn and milk

Immerse yourself completely in Mexican adventure by taking a tour around Tuxtla Gutiérrez.

A sip of chilled tequila during summer will totally refresh you!

VANCOUVER, CANADA

Mountainous Vancouver is a city in the province of British Columbia, known for having robust theater roots with lots of social and cultural diversity.

Vancouver's robust art and entertainment industry have national importance to Canada with regard to tourist attraction.

Vancouver has a current population of over 1 million people.

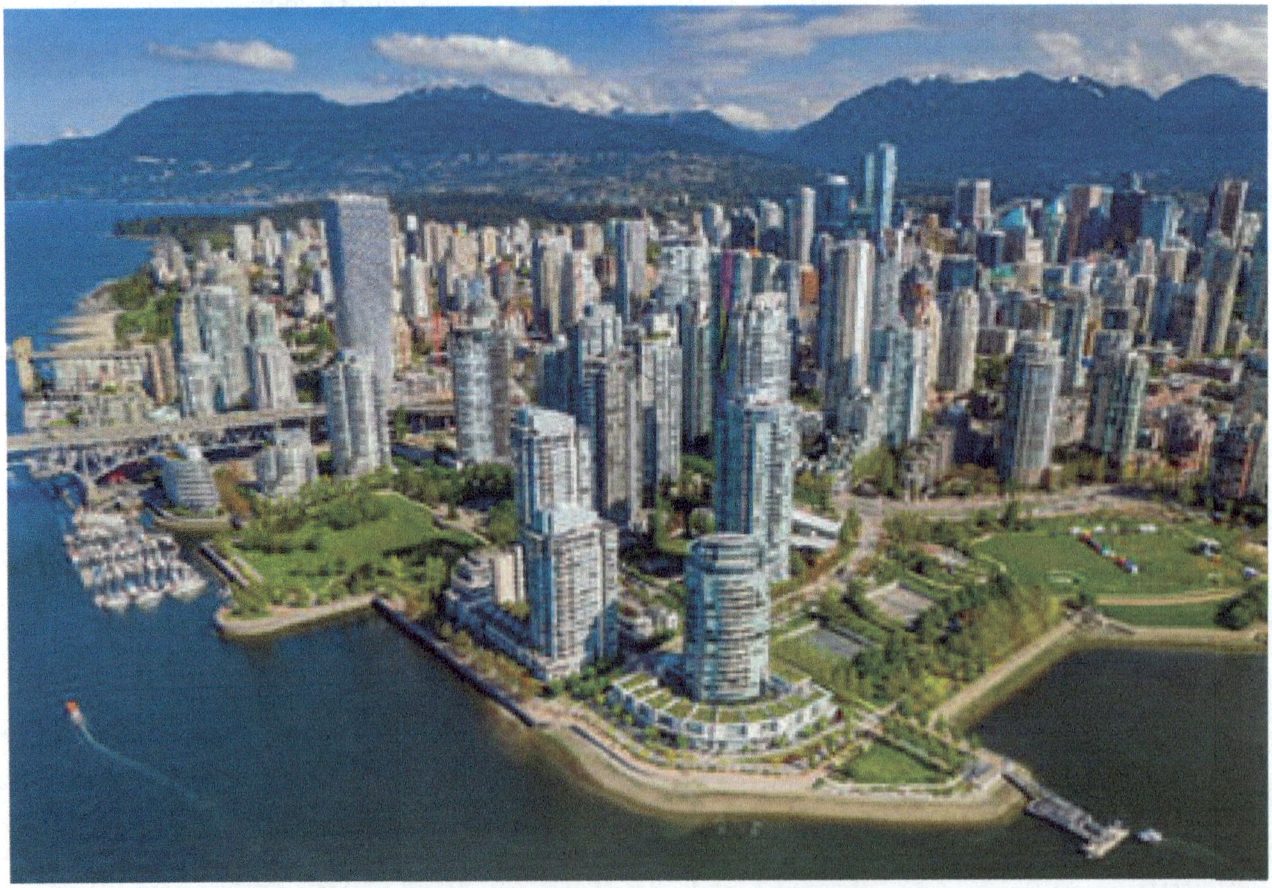

Raspberry Peach Soup

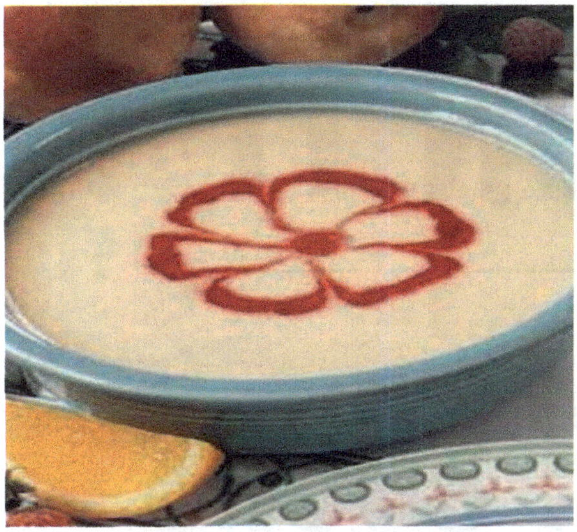

Amount of calories per serving is 100.

INGREDIENTS

- 2 cups water
- ¾ cup sugar
- 4 ounces (3 bunches) of fresh lemon-verbena leaves (about 4 cups or sprigs)
- ½ cup lime juice
- 4 medium yellow peaches
- ⅓ pint raspberries

Fruits are one of the best things about summer. Nothing else can taste as fresh and juicy as your summer staple fruits such as raspberries and peaches.
So, why not make them into a soup?

DIRECTIONS

1. In a medium saucepan, bring the water to a boil and add the sugar. Boil 2 minutes. Remove the pan from the heat, add all the lemon-verbena sprigs and submerge them completely in the sugar syrup. Cover and let cool down to room temperature. Add the lime juice and strain into a large bowl.
2. In a saucepan of boiling water, heat the peaches for 30 seconds. Transfer to a bowl of ice water and remove the skins. Working with one peach at a time, hold the peach in your hand and make thin slices to the stone all around the fruit. Gently flick off the slices into the sugar syrup with the knife.
3. Add the raspberries, cover and refrigerate for 1 hour.

Vancouver's Grouse Mountainmust try for lovers of heights.

SECTION 11

BREAKFAST SOUPS

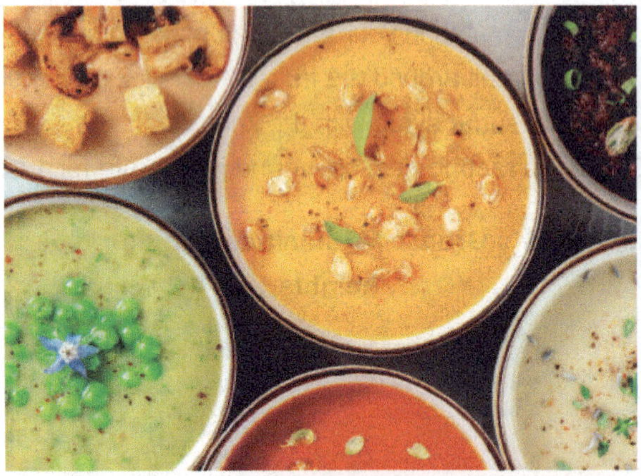
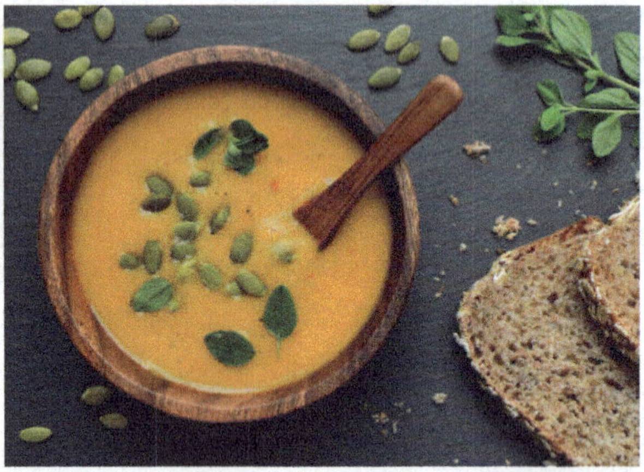
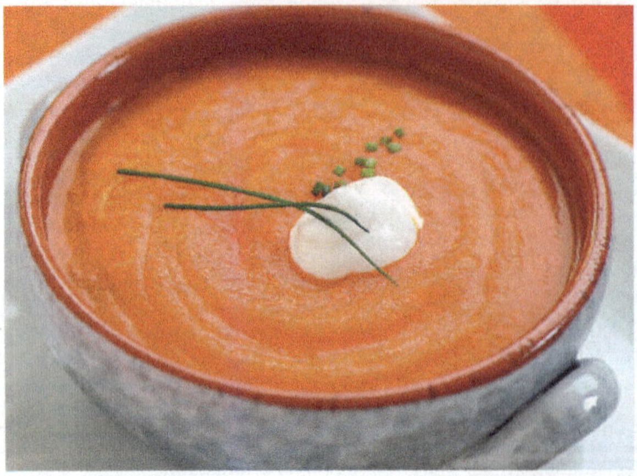
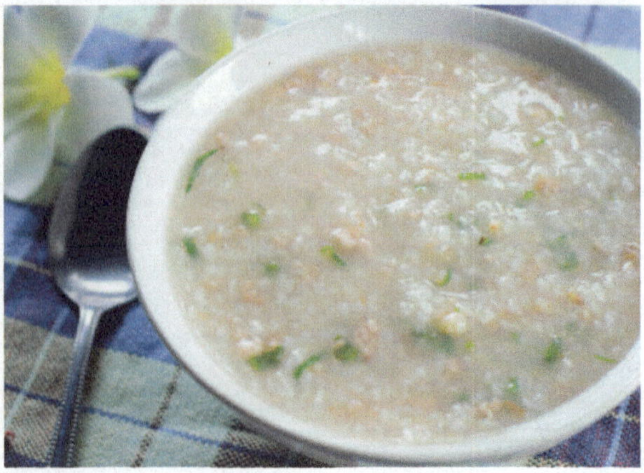

AFRICA

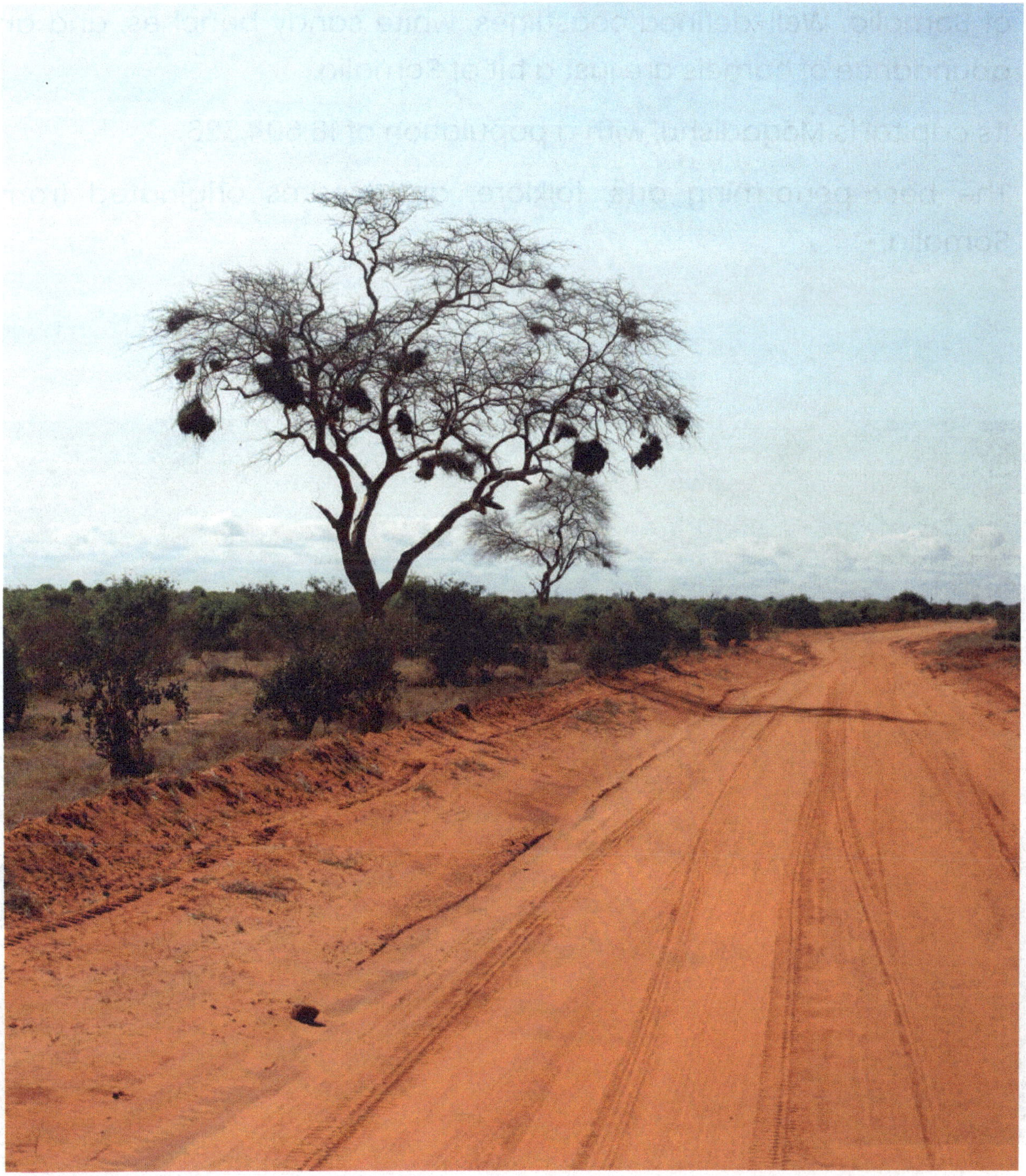

SOMALIA

The East African country is officially known as the Federal Republic of Somalia. Well-defined coastlines, white sandy beaches, and an abundance of camels are just a bit of Somalia.

Its capital is Mogadishu, with a population of 16,604,326.

The best performing arts, folklore, and poems originated from Somalia.

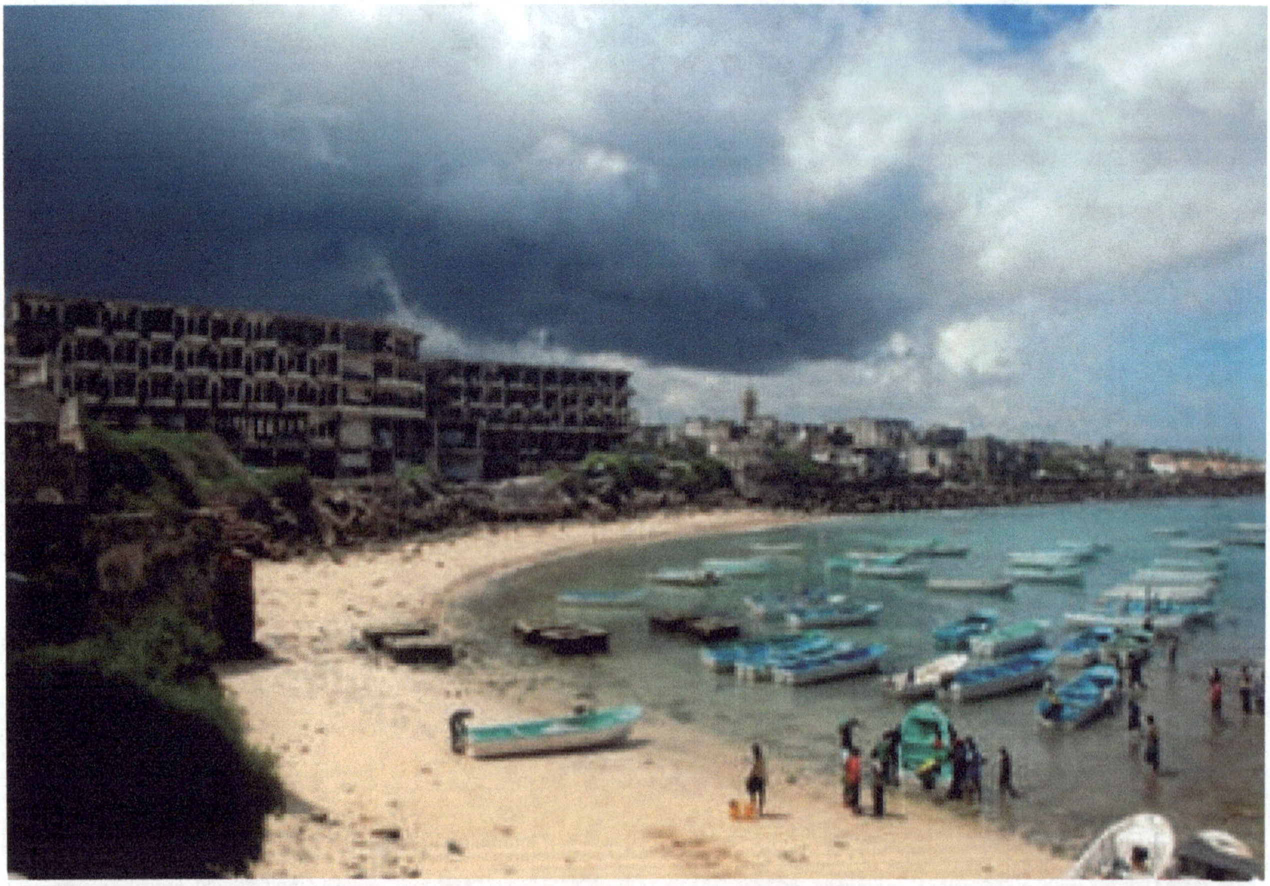

MaraqFahfah (Somali Soup)

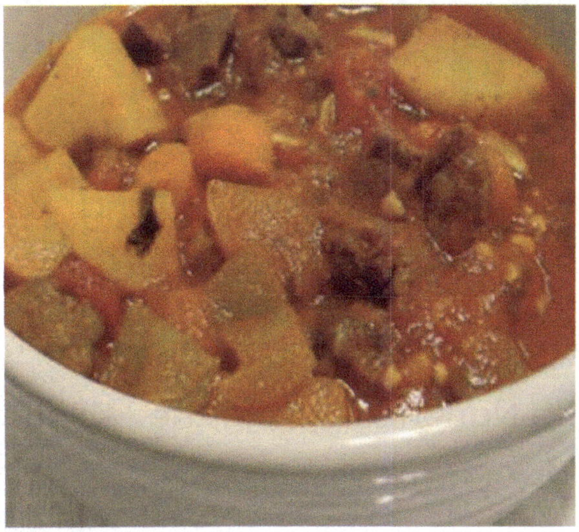

Amount of calories per serving is 245.

INGREDIENTS

- 2 pounds meat
- 1 sliced tomato
- 1 sliced small onion
- 2 minced garlic
- 2 tbsp coriander leaves
- 2 tsp ground coriander
- 1 green chili finely chopped
- juice of 1/2 lemon
- 2 bouillon cubes
- 1 cup water
- 3 medium potatoes
- 2 carrots chopped
- ¾ head of cabbage
- salt and ground pepper to taste

This traditional soup can be made with seafood. This MaraqFahfah meaty hearty soup has plenty of vegetables, and potatoes, flavored with chili, lemon juice, and coriander.

DIRECTIONS

1. Add the meat to a pan, crumble in the beef cubes then cover with water. Bring to a boil and cook for about 80 minutes, or until the meat is tender.
2. Add the potatoes, carrot, and cabbage then return to a simmer and cook for about 15 minutes before stirring in all the remaining vegetables. Season to taste then stir in the chili, lemon juice and coriander seeds. Return to a simmer, cover, and cook for about 20 minutes, or until the vegetables are tender.
3. Ladle into warmed serving bowls, garnish with coriander leaves and accompany with lahooh, rice, or bread.

Malawah pairs well with the SomalianMaraqFahfah.

LESOTHO

The South African country's state capital is Maseru and a population of over 2,169,522.

Breath-taking scenery which includes frosted hills.

You may wish to visit the Sehlabathebe National Park, in the Maloti Mountains which cream of vibrant biodiversity.

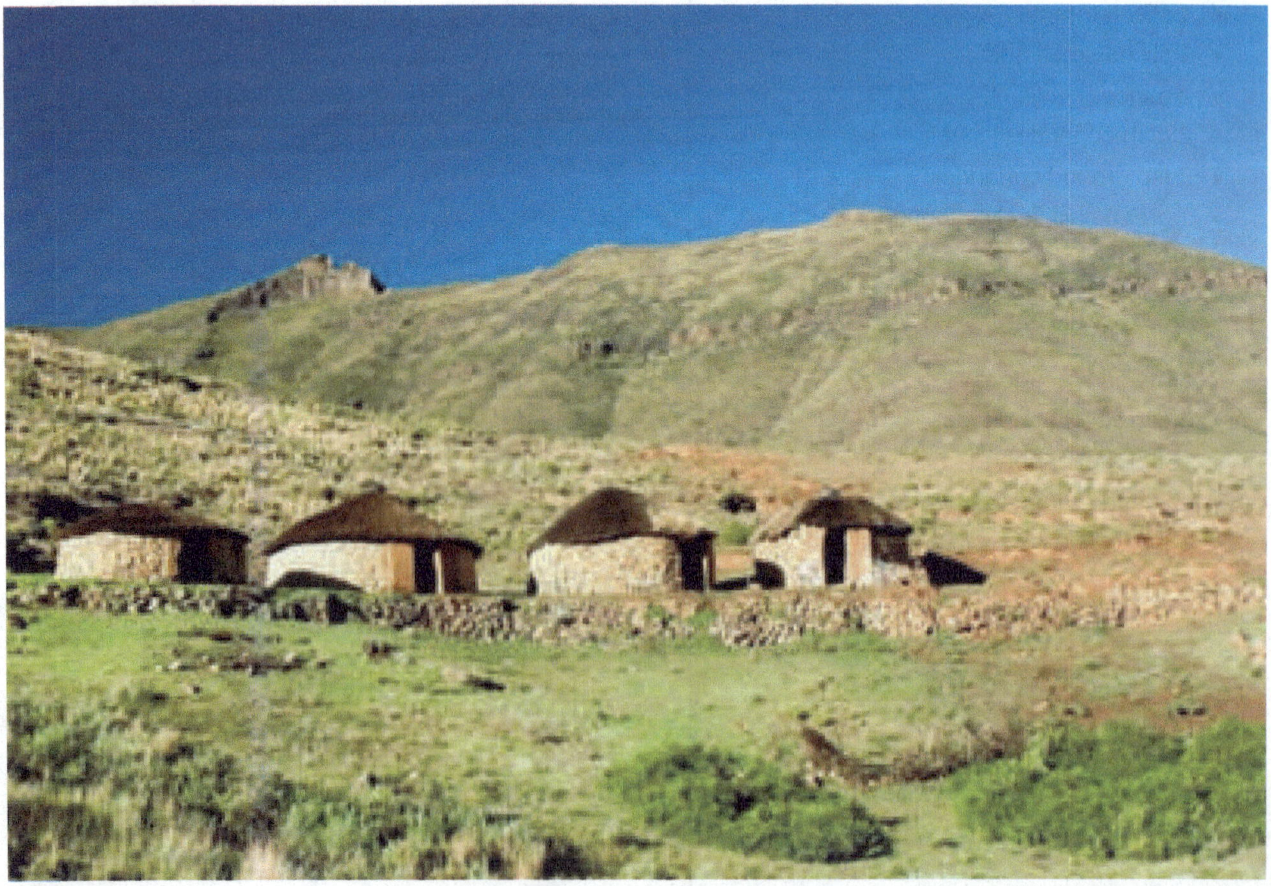

Spinach and Tangerine Soup (Butha-Buthe)

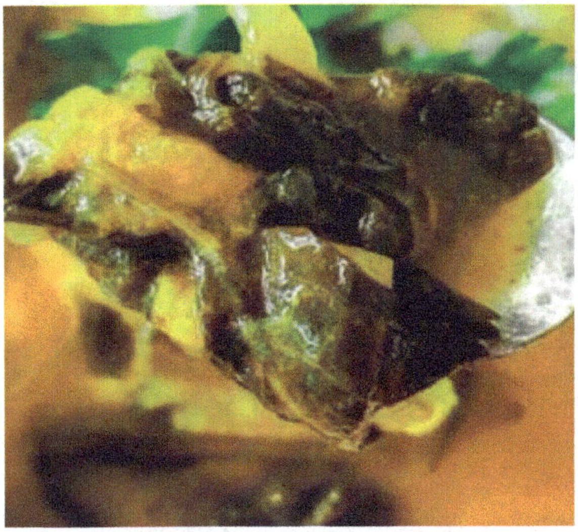

Amount of calories per serving is 136.8.

Spinach and tangerine soup is a traditional recipe from Lesotho that combines the sweetness and sourness of the citrus with the earthiness of spinach. It is enjoyed as breakfast.

INGREDIENTS

- 3 quarts chicken broth
- 3 onions , thinly sliced
- 1 lb fresh spinach , finely chopped
- ¾ cup yellow split peas
- 3 teaspoons turmeric powder
- ⅔ cup rice flour
- 4 tablespoons unsalted butter
- 2 lb tangerines (or mandarins)
- 1 bunch flat parsley , finely chopped
- 1 bunch cilantro , finely chopped
- 2 cups plain yogurt

DIRECTIONS

1. The day before, rinse the split peas and soak them in a large bowl of cold water.
2. The next day, bring the chicken broth to a boil in a large pot.
3. Rinse and drain the split peas and add them to a pot with the simmering chicken broth. Cover and cook over high heat for 20 minutes. Add boiling water if necessary, if the level is below the initial level.
4. Add the butter in a pan and sauté the onions for 5 minutes over medium heat until translucent.
5. Sprinkle turmeric on the onions and stir constantly over low heat for one minute.
6. Dilute the rice flour into ½ cup (150ml) of cold water and stir, then add this mixture to the onions and stir well. Pour this mixture immediately into the chicken broth.
7. Add the spinach, parsley, half of the cilantro, the zest of 2 tangerines (or mandarins) and the juice of four.
8. Cook for 20 minutes over low heat, stirring regularly.
9. Serve in individual bowls and pour 2 tablespoons of yogurt in the middle of the bowl and lightly sprinkle with cilantro.

ALGERIA

This North African country has a very large expanse of land, hence it's the largest African nation.

The capital of Algeria is Algiers.

Touring this nation will be a great idea considering their level of hospitality towards foreigners.

Algeria's land mass and human population seem to have a correlation; with 45,121,884 people.

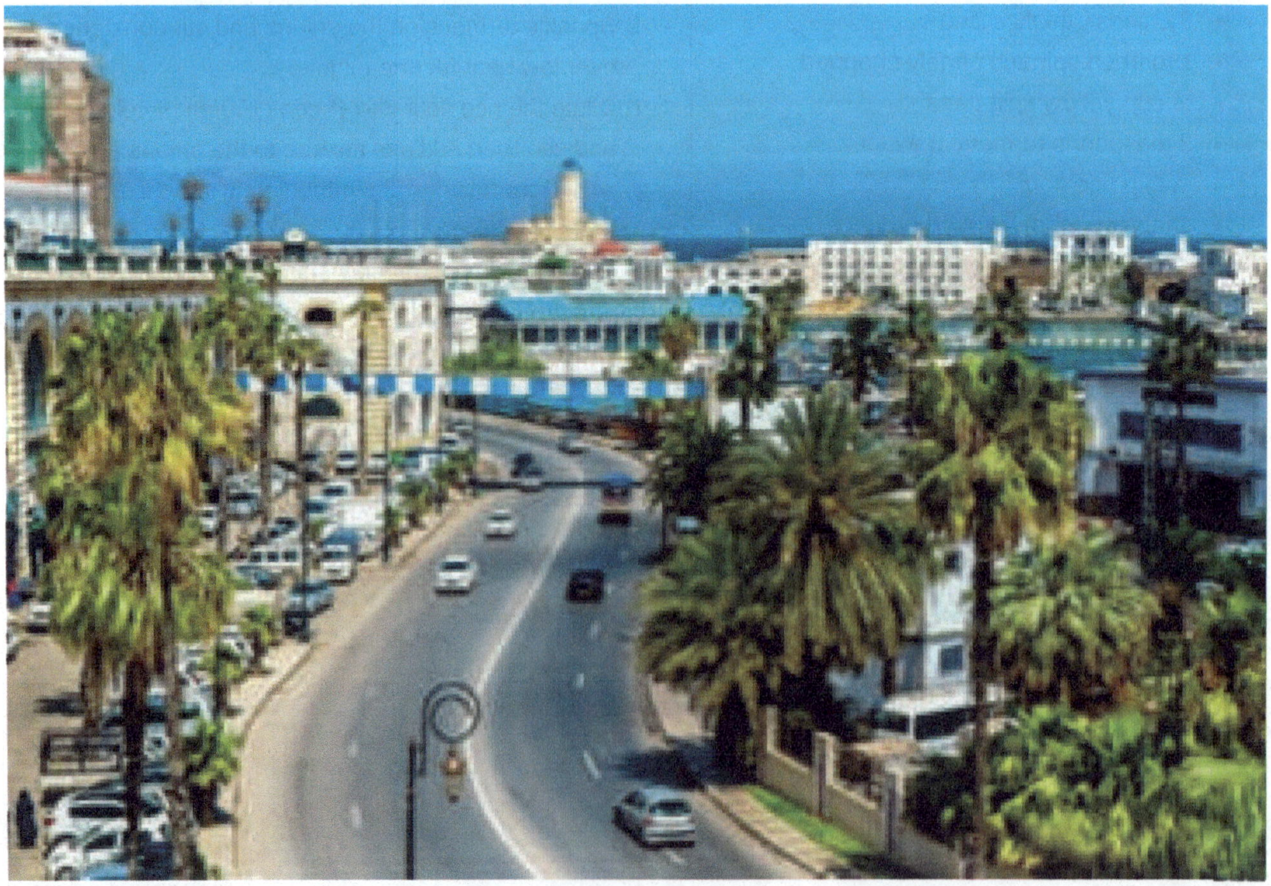

Algerian Chickpea Soup (Chorba / Shorba)

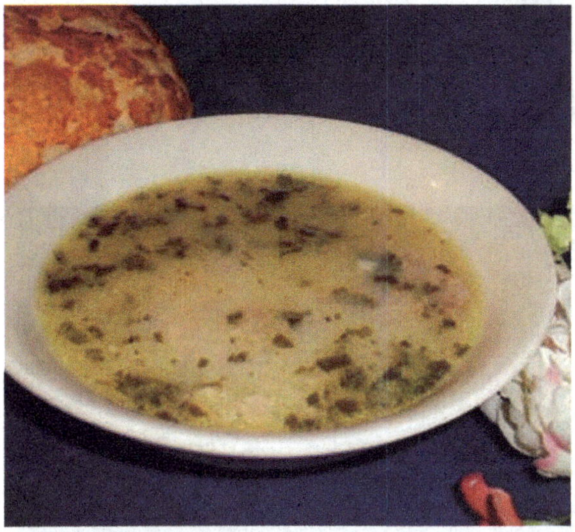

Amount of calories per serving is 143.

INGREDIENTS

- 1 -2 tablespoon olive oil
- 3 -4 chicken drumsticks
- 1 large onion, finely chopped
- 2 -3 garlic cloves, minced
- 4 teaspoons ras el hanout spice mix
- 1/2 teaspoon ginger
- 1/2 teaspoon turmeric
- 1/4 teaspoon cinnamon
- 3/4 teaspoon sweet paprika
- 1 liter chicken stock
- 1 liter of water
- 500 g canned chickpeas
- 400 g chopped canned tomatoes
- 1/4 preserved lemon, very finely chopped
- 1/4 cup fresh cilantro, chopped
- 1/2 lemon juice
- 1-2 tablespoon olive oil

Delicious Chickpea Soup is a flavorful Algerian dish that can be enjoyed for breakfast!

DIRECTIONS

1. Place oil in a large pan, add the chicken & fry to seal all over. Add the spices & fry for a minute more.
2. Add all the other ingredients except the coriander/cilantro, chickpeas & lemon juice. Bring to a boil then reduce heat, cover & simmer 1 hour.
3. Add the chickpeas to the pan. Take the chicken from the pan & remove all the meat from the bones, shred & put back into the pan. Simmer for a further 20 minutes.
4. If the soup is the consistency you like, you can add the coriander/ cilantro & lemon juice now. Simmer for 1 minute, re-season if desired & then serve.
5. If you feel the soup needs to be a little thicker, you can eitherreduce it by cooking furtheror thicken with it plain flour.

Oran, Constantine are other cities to sample for a feel of Algeria

ASIA

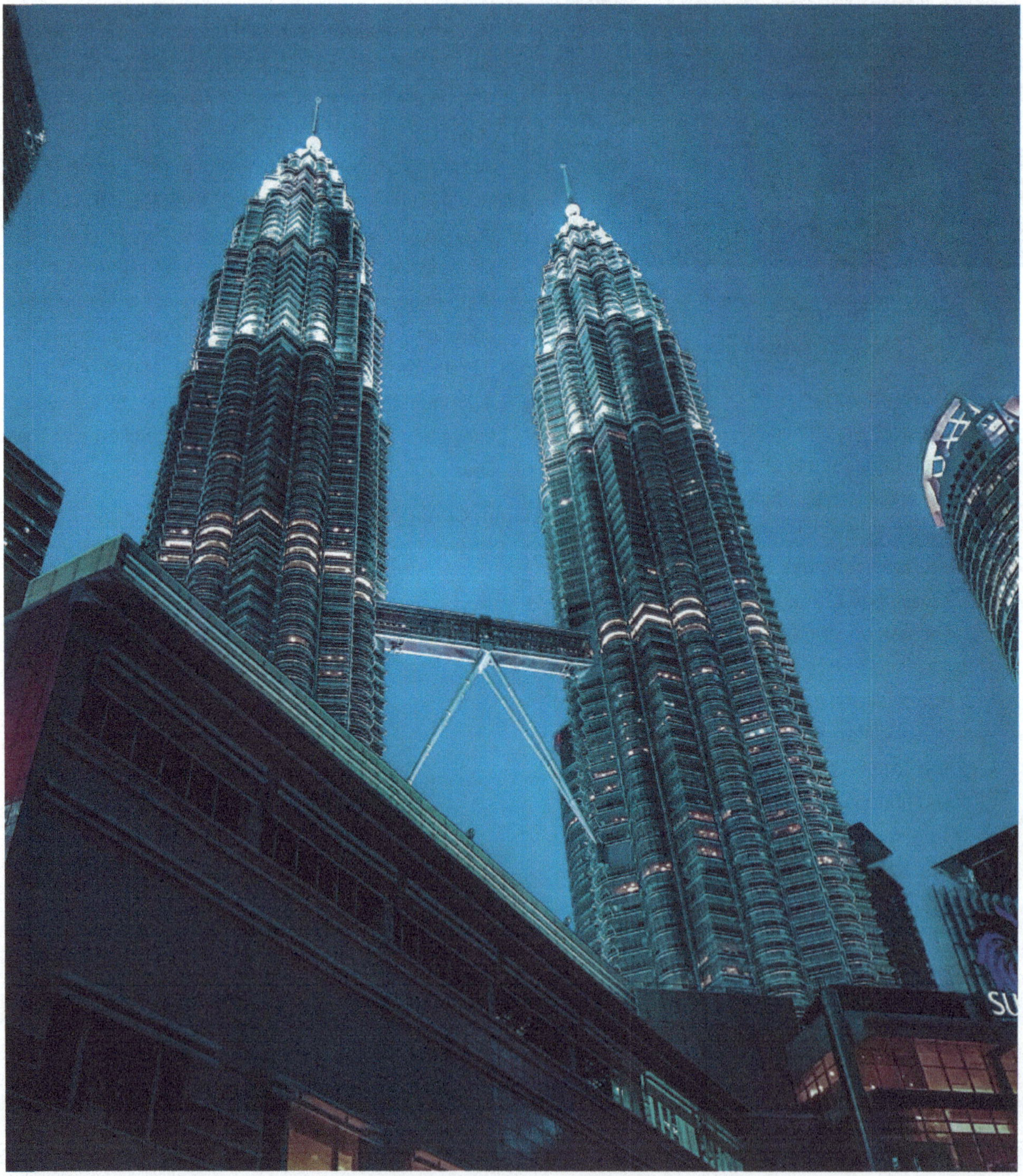

SYRIA

Does Golan heights ring a bell?

This West Asian country is also known as the Syrian Arab Republic.

The capital of Syria is Damascus.
Economically relevant forest produce, rich cultural heritage and social diversity are part and parcel of Syria

Damask fabric was so named, bearing its roots in Damascus (fondly called the pearl of the East, and commercial hub of Syria).

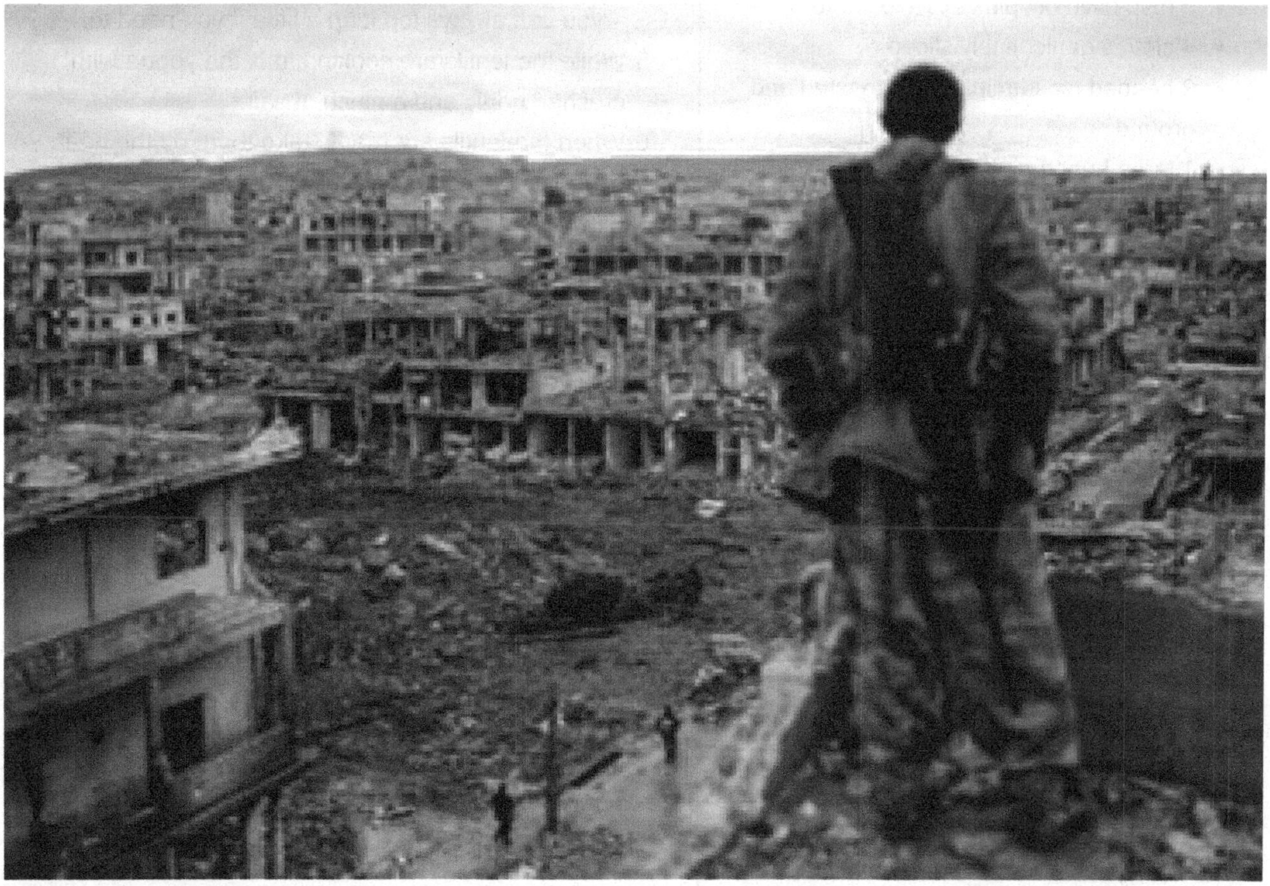

Syrian Lentil Soup

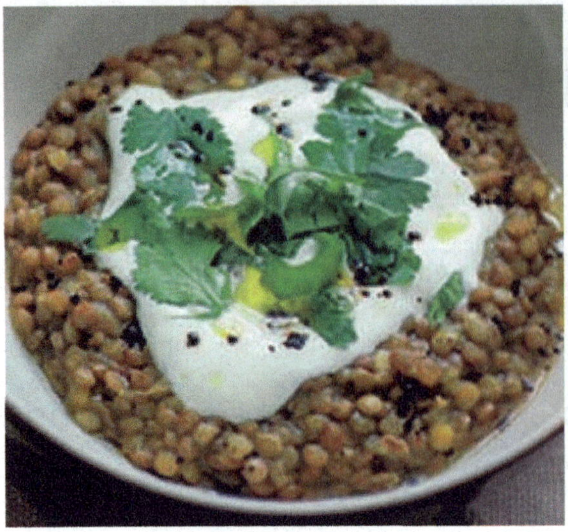

A hearty lentil soup is also called Addes. This nutritious soup is simple and easy to prepare.

INGREDIENTS

- 300 g lentils (green or brown)
- 3 medium onions, finely sliced
- 3 tbsp olive oil, plus extra to serve
- 4 cloves garlic, finely sliced
- 3 heaped tsp cumin seeds, toasted and ground
- 1 large bunch fresh coriander (stalks and leaves separated)
- 1 3/4 liters of cold water
- 4 tbsp Greek yogurt
- 1/2 clove garlic, crushed
- salt
- juice of ½ a lemon
- chili flakes

DIRECTIONS

1. Soak the lentils in a bowl of cold water, rinsing them several times to remove any dirt or grit.
2. Over moderate heat, cook the onions in the oil for a good 10 minutes. You want them soft and beginning to turn golden.
3. Add the garlic and toasted cumin and continue to fry over moderate heat for another couple of minutes.
4. Add the coriander stalks and the water, or enough to fully cover the lentil mix. Turn up the heat and bring to a boil. Skim off any froth that surfaces. Turn the temperature down and continue to cook at a moderate bubble for about 30 minutes, watching the water level – you can always top it up a little if you need to.
5. While the lentils are cooking, mix the yogurt with crushed garlic and a pinch of salt.
6. When the lentils are ready, take them off the heat. You want the individual lentils to be completely squishable between two fingers and the whole to be a soupy mass.
7. Taste the lentils and add salt as needed. Add the lemon juice.
8. Serve the lentils in bowls and to each add a spoonful of seasoned yoghurt, some coriander leaves, a sprinkle of chili flakes and a spoonful of olive oil.
9. We like to eat this with warm flatbreads, to mop up the lentils.

Consider taking a trip around The Greatest Crusader Fortress in the World or visit the Beehive Houses at Al Jaboul Lake.

QATAR

The Middle East Arab country with a population of over 2,959,276 has its capital in Doha.

It holds very large depots of oil and gas.

Qatar has a taxless, yet buoyant economy.

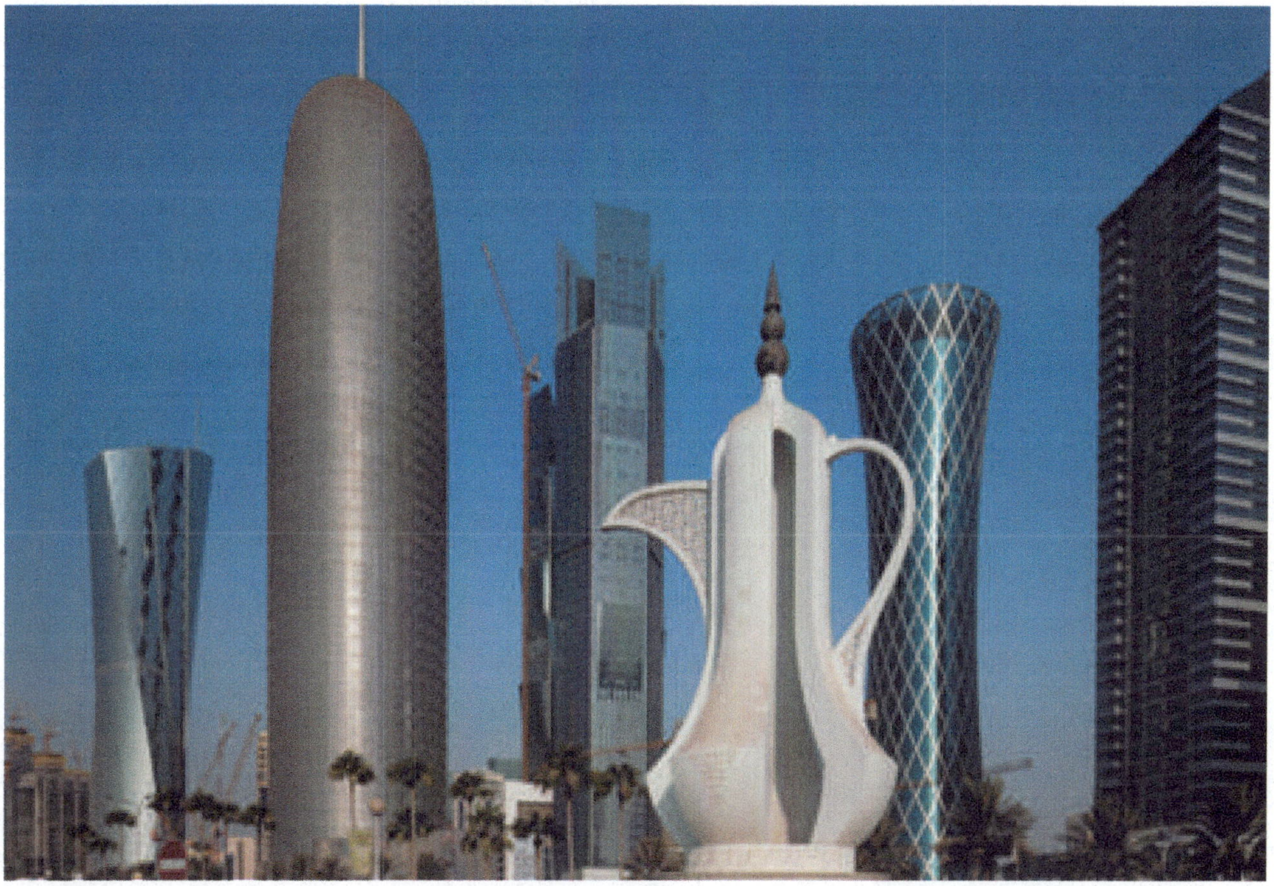

Qatari Lentil Soup

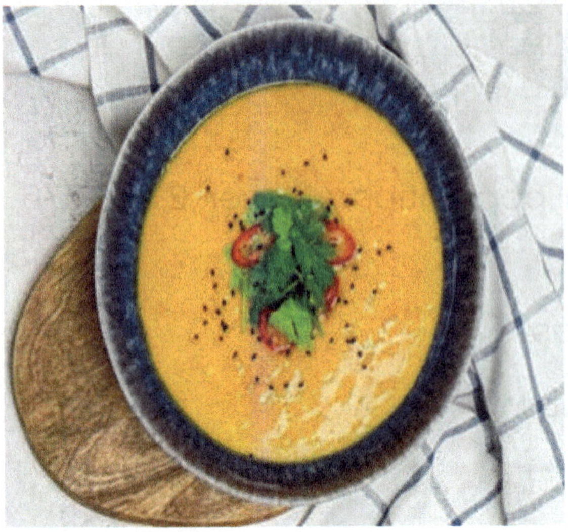

INGREDIENTS

- Celery (chopped) 80 g
- Carrots (julienned) 120 g
- Yellow lentil 300 g
- Vegetable stock 1.5 l
- Onion (sliced) 100 g
- Potato (cubed) 250 g
- White pepper powder 1 g
- Cumin powder 2 g
- Corn oil40 g
- Salt 12 g

Balaleet is a traditional Ramadan savory dish popular in the Arab states of the Persian Gulf.

A popular breakfast choice, it traditionally consists of many natural ingredients.

DIRECTIONS

Prepare the lentils

1. Rinse and drain the lentils.
2. Heat oil and sauté onion, celery, potatoes, and carrots for three minutes until softened.
3. Add the lentils and stir for five minutes.
4. Add salt, pepper, and cumin and stir for a minute.
5. Add vegetable stock and bring to a boil.

Make the soup

1. Reduce heat and simmer for 35 minutes or until the lentils are cooked.
2. Blend the lentils into a smooth mixture with a hand blender.
3. Season to taste.
4. Serve with fried or toasted Arabic bread pieces and lemon wedges.

Seeking to relax completely in Qatar?

A tour of the Banana Islands will surely take your breath away!

How about unwinding slowly on the Fuwairit Beach?

OCEANIA

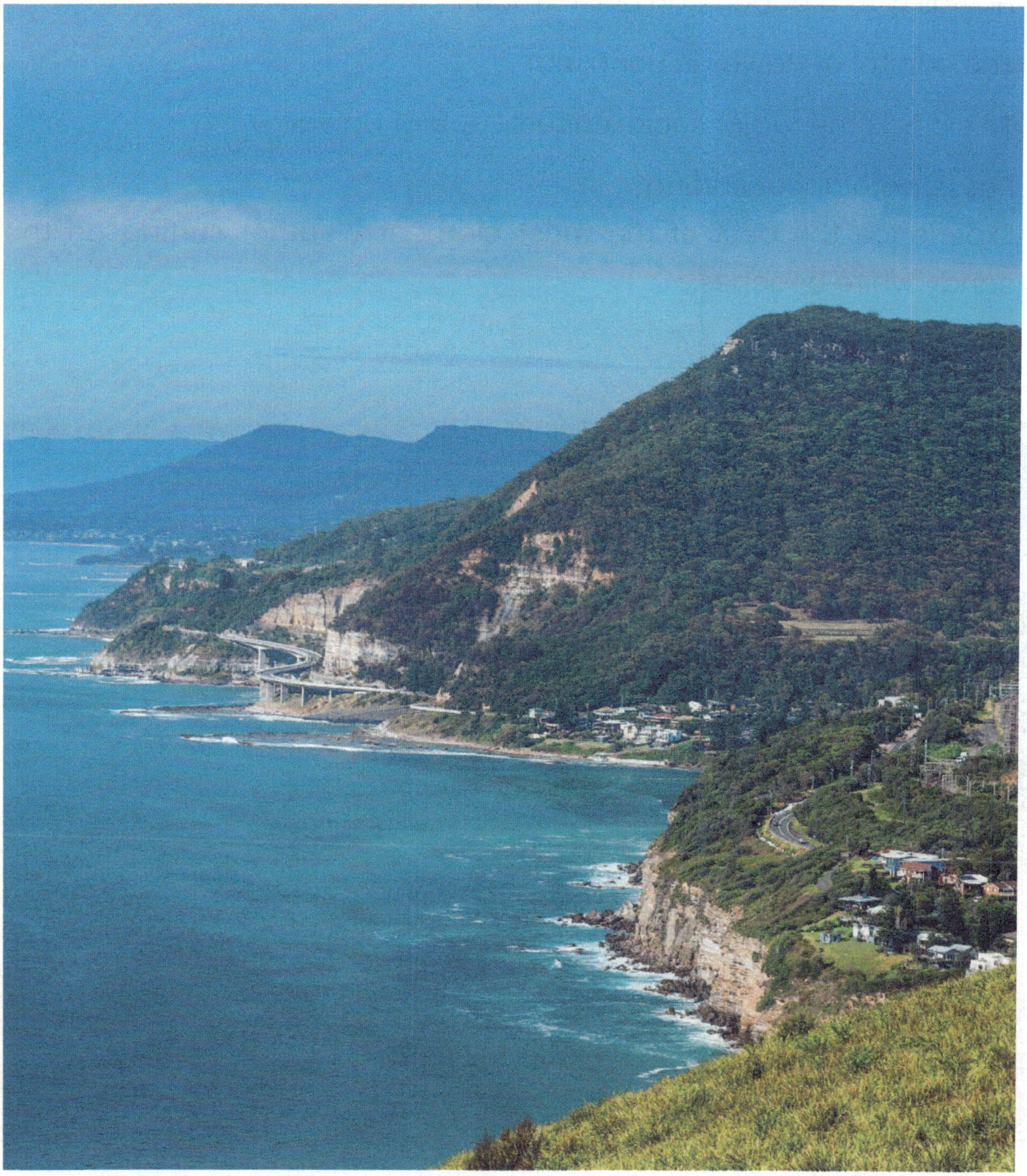

HAWAII

Hawaii with a population of 1,433,336.

The capital of Hawaii is Honolulu.

This city is the major socio-cultural hub of Hawaii.

Passionate about surfing?
Experience the best of the most clement weather surfing on the sandy white beaches.

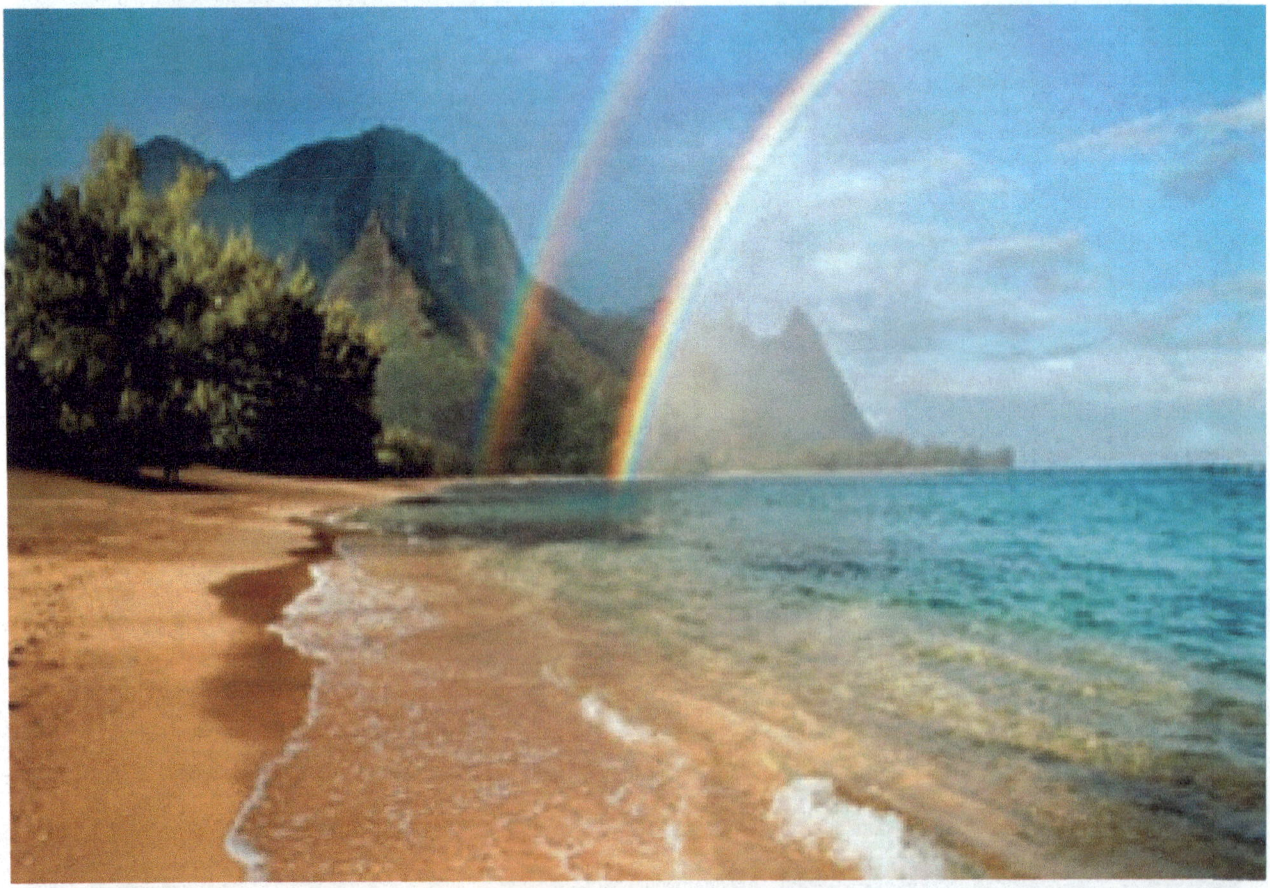

Hawaiian Saimin Noddle Soup

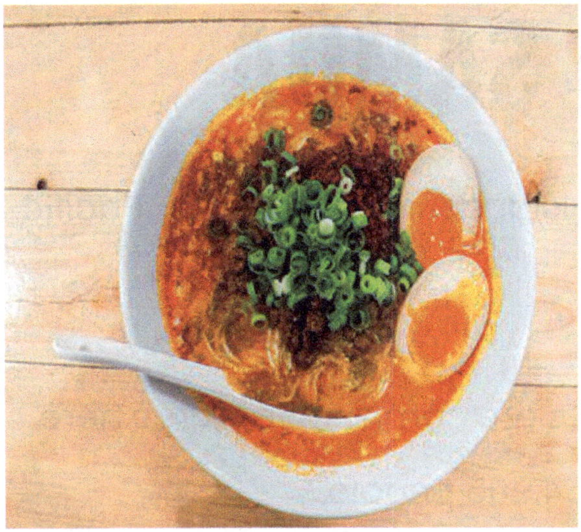

Made from eggs noodles and wheat. Saimin is a popular noodles meal in Hawaii.

INGREDIENTS

Noodles

- 2 bundles of saimin noodles (fresh or frozen)

Quick Broth

- 4 cups chicken broth
- 2 teaspoons dashi powder
- 1 tablespoon soy sauce
- 1 1-inch knob of ginger, smashed

Toppings

- Spam thinly sliced
- Scrambled egg, thinly sliced
- Kamaboko (fishcake), sliced
- Green onions, chopped

DIRECTIONS

1. Make the broth. Bring the chicken broth to a boil, then add in the dashi powder, soy sauce, and ginger. Simmer the broth for 15-30 minutes.
2. Boil the saimin noodles according to package instructions. Drain and divide between two bowls.
3. Pour the broth over the noodles. Add the toppings.
4. Eat hot and enjoy!

AMERICAN SAMOA

American Samoa boasts of many Islands in the South Pacific region.

The largest Island is in Pago.

Coral reefs, beaches, and green forests are common features here.

This region boasts of a population of 54,995 people.

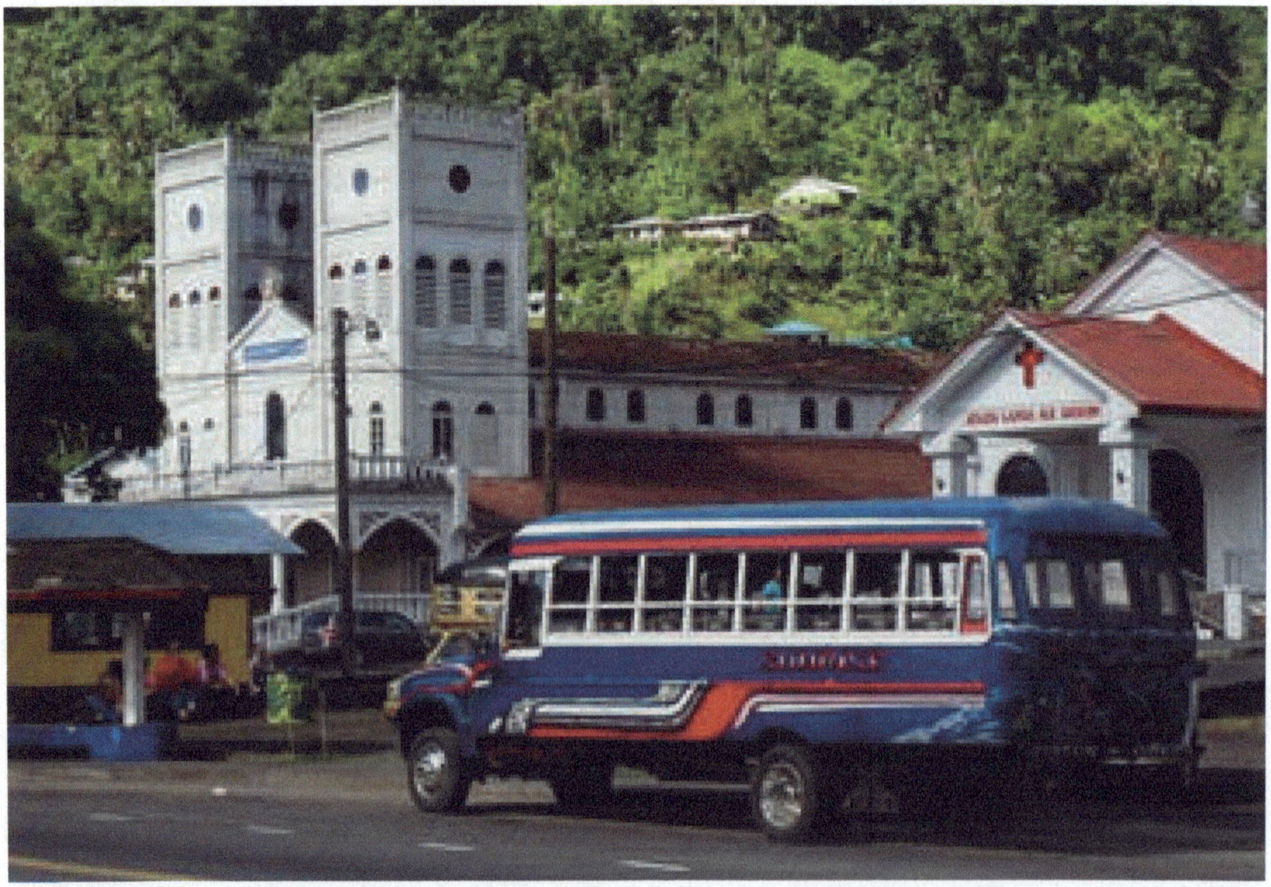

Samoan Banana Soup

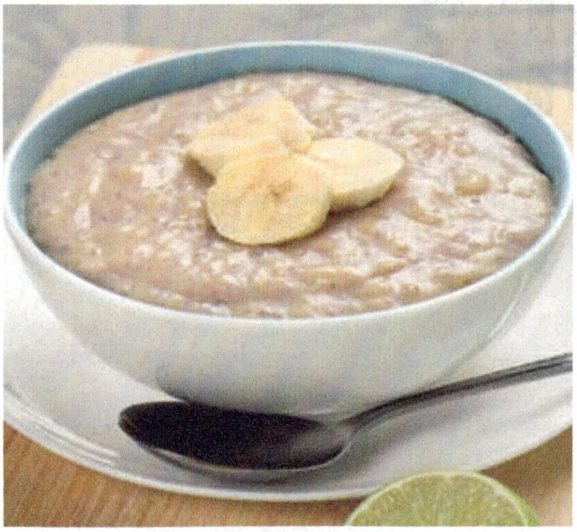

Amount of calories per serving is 137.

INGREDIENTS

- 2 ripe bananas
- 1 cup water
- 2-3 tbsp tapioca pearls (sabudana)
- ¼ – ⅓ cup coconut milk
- 1-2 tsp sugar -optional

This perfect Samoan soup serves well as breakfast, lunch or dinner!! Perfect with nice hot bread & butter. A taste of this will leave you speechless!

DIRECTIONS

1. Soak the tapioca pearls in water for 30 minutes.
2. Slice the bananas and add to a pan. Add the water.
3. Put the pan on medium heat.
4. Let the banana cook in the water till it becomes soft.
5. Mash the cooked banana lightly with a masher or a fork.
6. Add the tapioca pearls and let the mixture simmer till the tapioca pearls are cooked. They should become transparent. Remember to stir the mixture occasionally so that the tapioca pearls do not stick to the bottom of the pan.
7. When the tapioca is done, add coconut milk.
8. Let the mixture become hot and serve immediately.

A visit to Nu'uuli Falls will make you do a come-back to visit the Samoans!

EUROPE

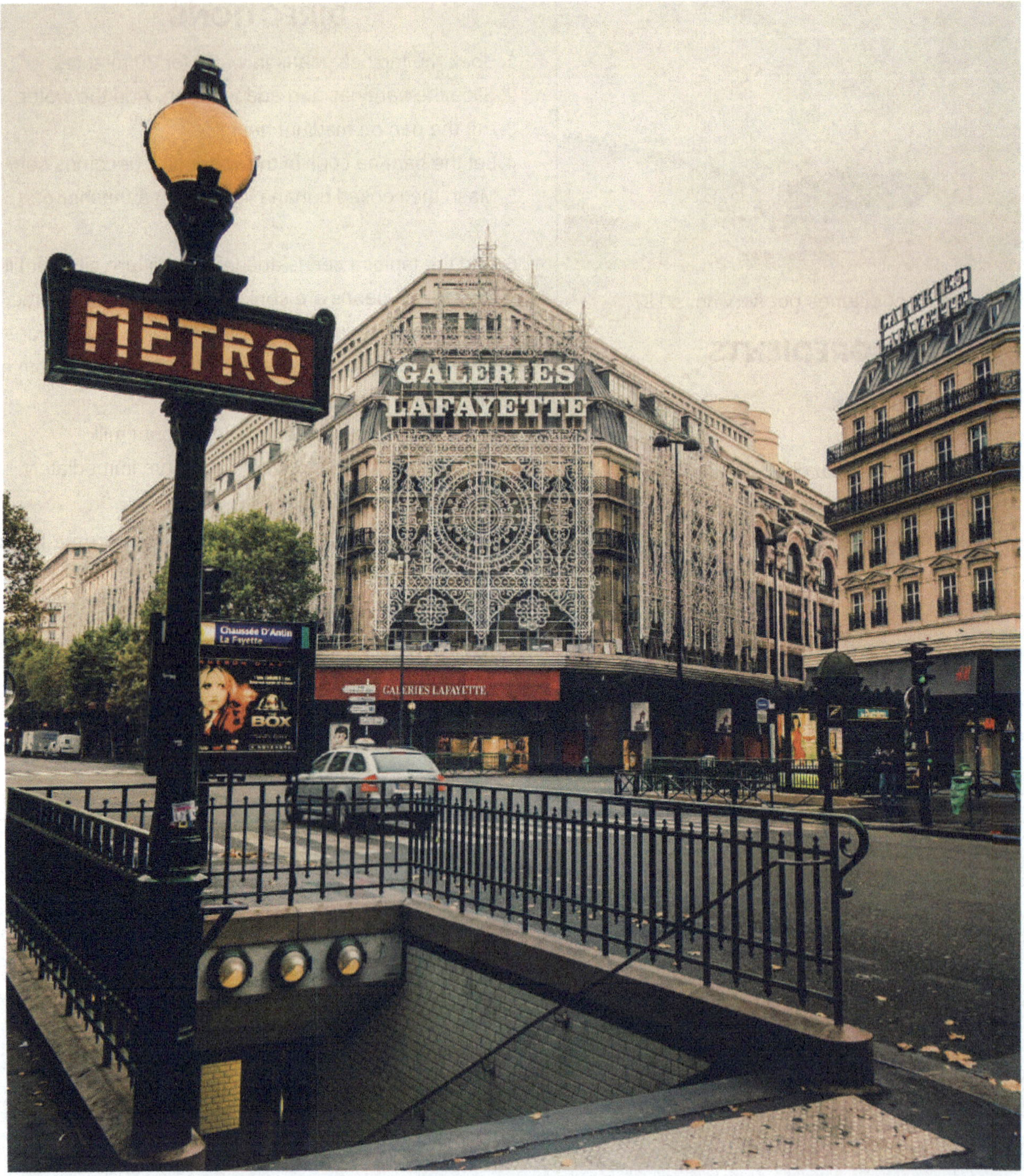
METRO
GALERIES
LAFAYETTE
Chaussée D'Antin
La Fayette
BOX
GALERIES LAFAYETTE

BELARUS

The capital of this Eastern Europe country is Minsk.

It has a population of 9,444,300.

This country is also called the 'Lungs of Europe'.

The best potatoes can be found in this country.

Nightlife music and dance are commonplace on the streets of this country.

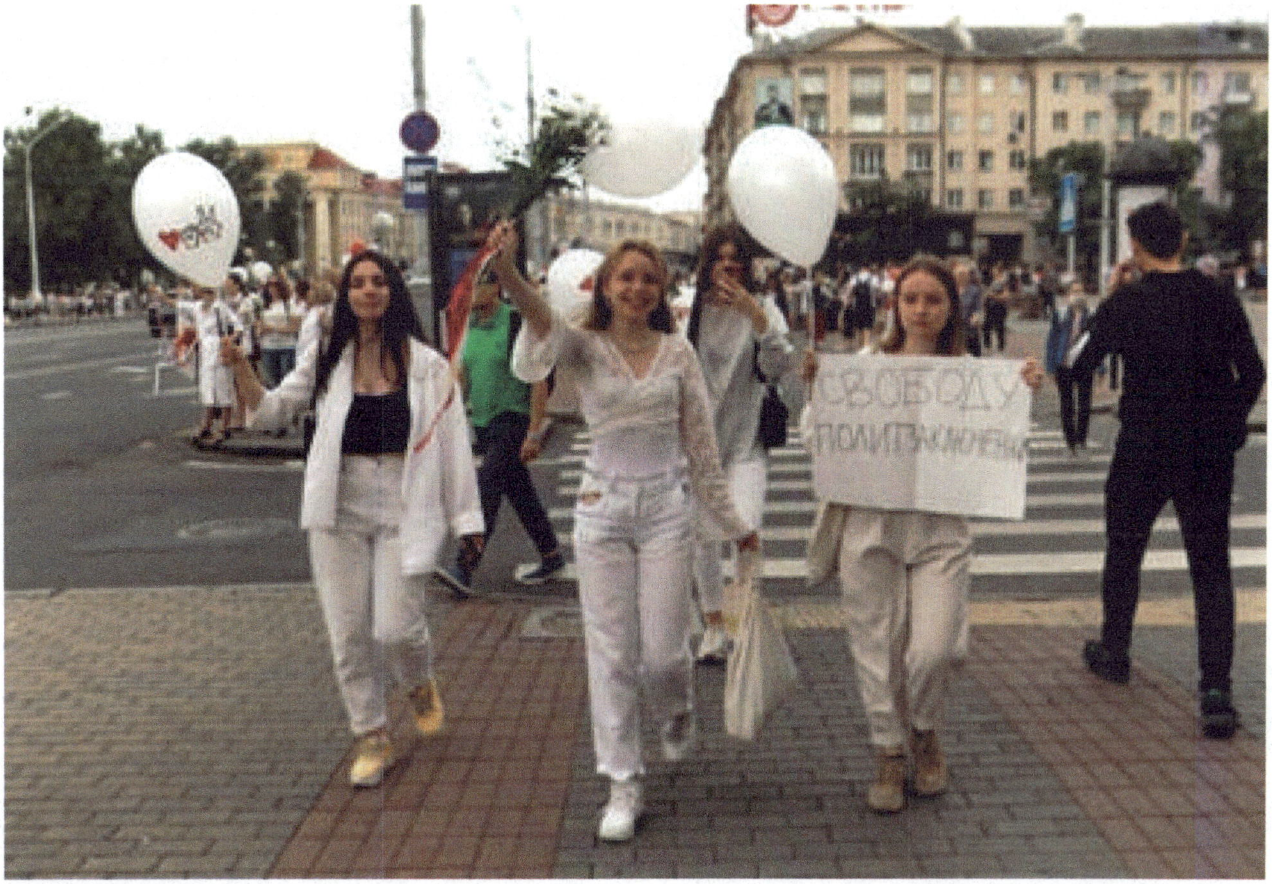

Borscht Belarusian Soup

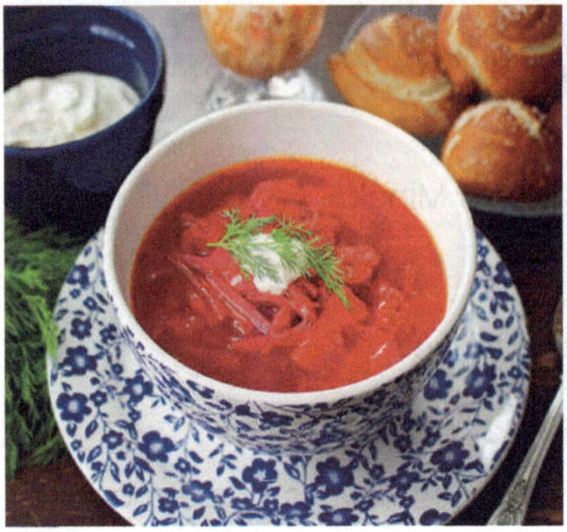

This main ingredient is beet which imparts that rich red color.
It is a traditional dish of East Slavs (Russia, Ukraine and Belarus) and a unique Belarus dish.

INGREDIENTS

- 24 oz (680 g) homemade vegetables and chicken broth, or the type of broth you prefer
- 14,6 oz (415 g) water
- 10,5 oz (300 g) raw beet, peeled and cut into small squares
- 15,5 oz (440 g) veal shank + 2 Tbsp olive oil
- 1 large red potato, 350 g approximately, cut into small squares
- 3,5 oz (100 g) red onion, finely chopped
- 2 large carrots, peeled and cut into small squares
- 2 large garlic cloves, minced
- 10,5 oz (300 g) red cabbage, shredded, use a mandolin
- 1 big red tomato, diced in small squares
- 4 Tbsp olive oil
- 2 Tbsp dark muscovado sugar
- 2 Tbsp apple cider vinegar
- 1 tsp coriander seeds
- 2 bay leaves
- salt and pepper to taste

For Garnish:

- crème fraîche
- fresh dill
- fresh parsley

DIRECTIONS

1. Cook the veal shank.
2. In a large saucepan pour 2 tablespoons of olive oil and place in a medium-high heat.
3. Once the temperature is taken, but be careful not to burn the oil and start smoking, add the veal shank. Cook on both sides until it gets a nice golden color, it will take between 2-3 minutes.
4. Season with salt and pepper, add the broth, reduce to medium low heat and cook, with the lid on leaving a little opening, for 1 hour and 30 minutes or 1 hour and 45 minutes. Or until the meat is very tender.
5. Turn off the heat, remove the meat and cut into small pieces or shred, according to our choice.
6. Add it back to the broth, set aside with the pot covered.

LATVIA

Perhaps, a visit to Riga's Central Market (one of Europe's biggest markets) will make you rethink marketing.

Latvia is a country on the Baltic Sea between Lithuania and Estonia.

Its landscape is marked by wide beaches as well as dense, sprawling forests.

Latvia's capital is Riga.

Latvia has a population of about 1,852,641 persons and is home to Europe's widest waterfall.

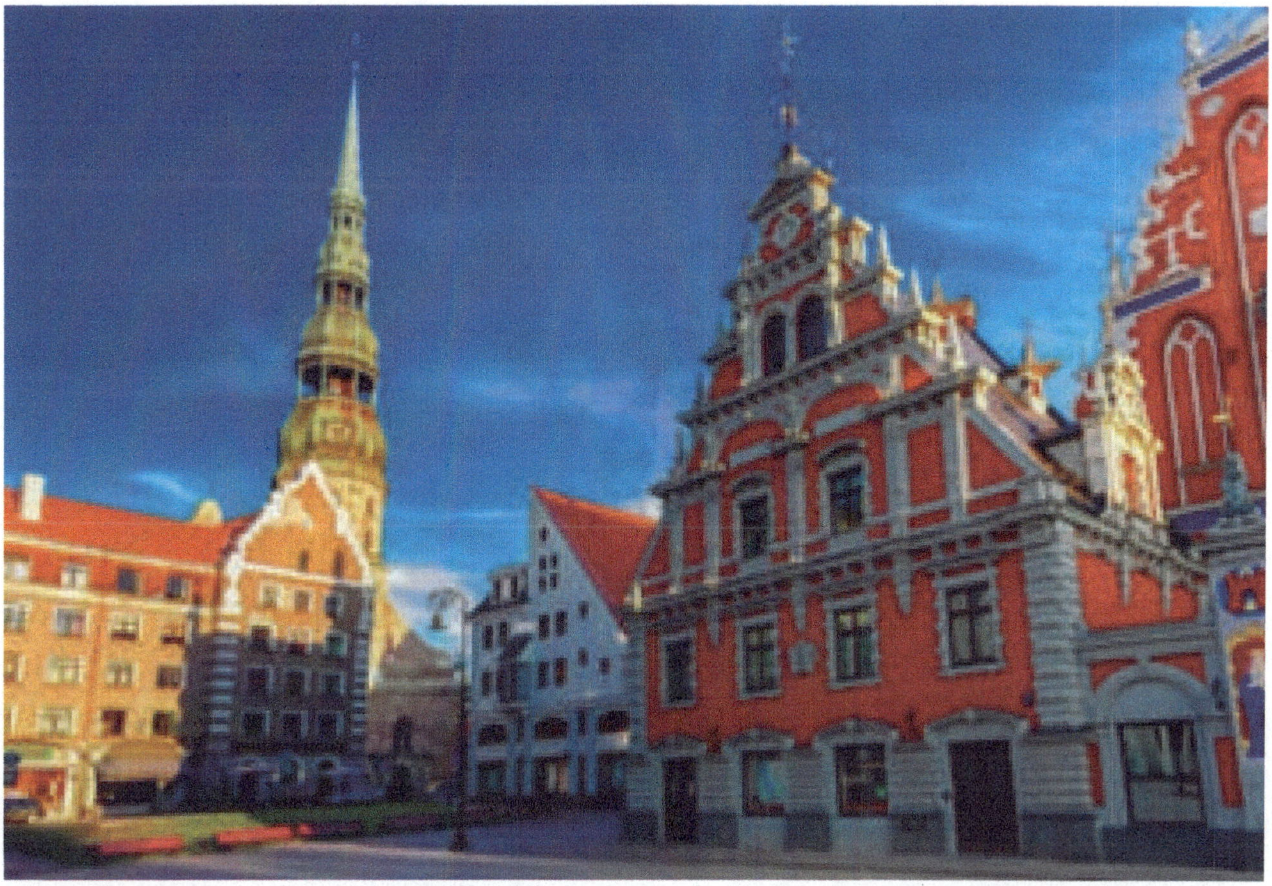

Latvian Cold Beet Soup

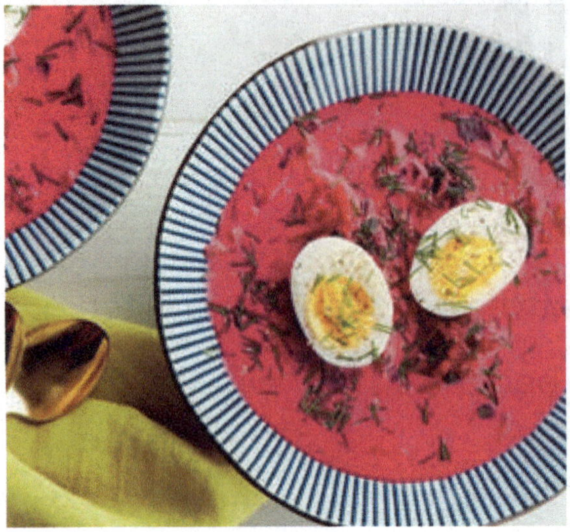

Amount of calories per serving is 202kcal

INGREDIENTS

- 2 small cooked beets
- 2 small cucumbers
- 4 large boiled eggs
- 4 tablespoons finely chopped dill
- 2 green onion
- 6 radishes
- 3 cups kefir (or more for a thinner soup)
- Lots of salt

Cold Beet Soup is a healthy soup for summer. This creamy soup is prepared with cucumbers, eggs, sweet beets, and kefir will leave you coming back for more.

It's simple and hearty, making use of what is on hand.

DIRECTIONS

1. Grate the cooked beets.
2. Finely chop the rest of the ingredients.
3. Add all the chopped and grated ingredients to a bowl.
4. Pour kefir over the ingredients and mix.
5. Add enough salt to taste.
6. Eat cold.

Latvia is a sure place to sample the wonders of nature in forestry!

NORWAY

Historic mountains, greenery, and landscapes.

Norway has a record for hiking and skiing.

The Nordic European country has a population of over 6 million people.

Ever thought of beholding the Norwegian salmon? You are just in luck!

Norwegian breakfast meals feature a variety of bread types.

Whole grain bread are commonly served at breakfast.

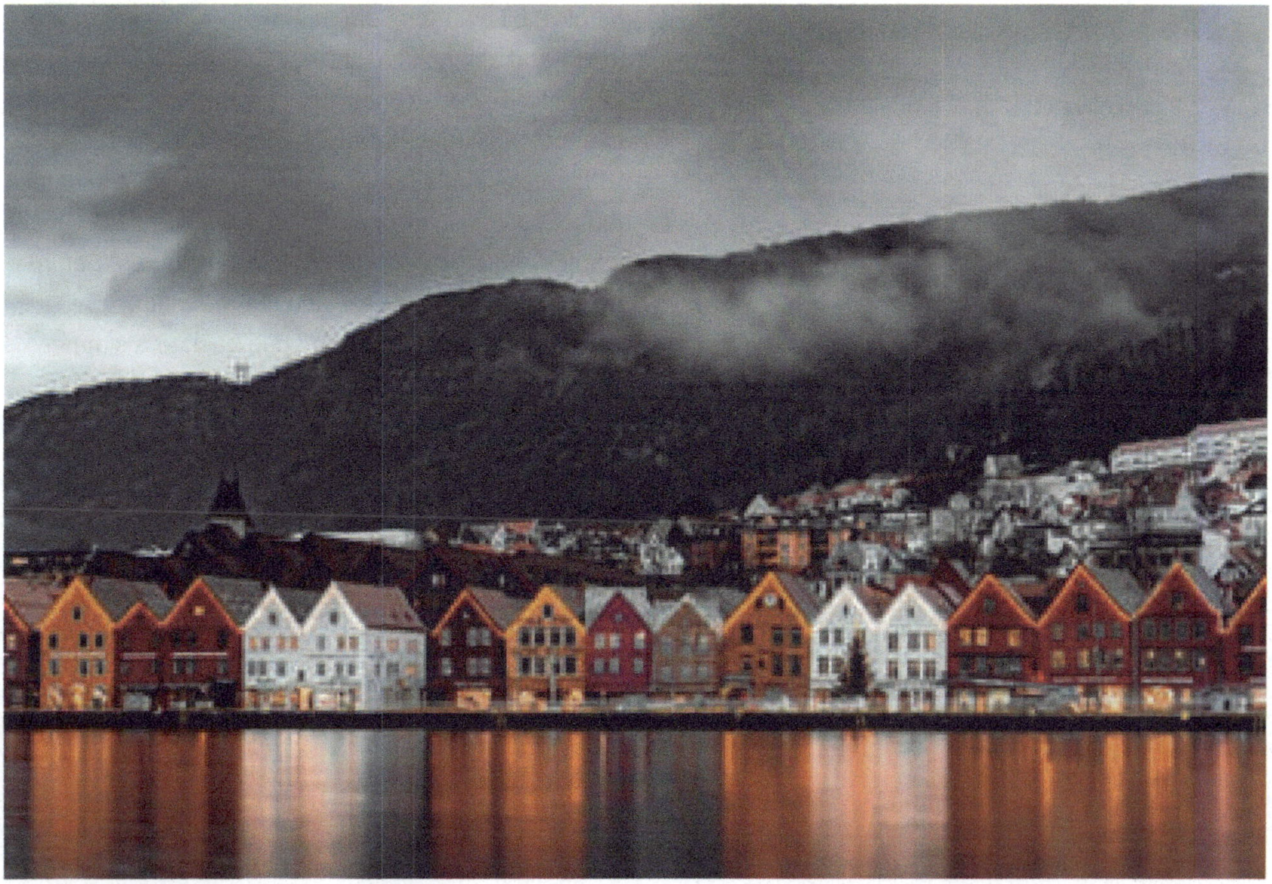

Norwegian Fiskesuppe

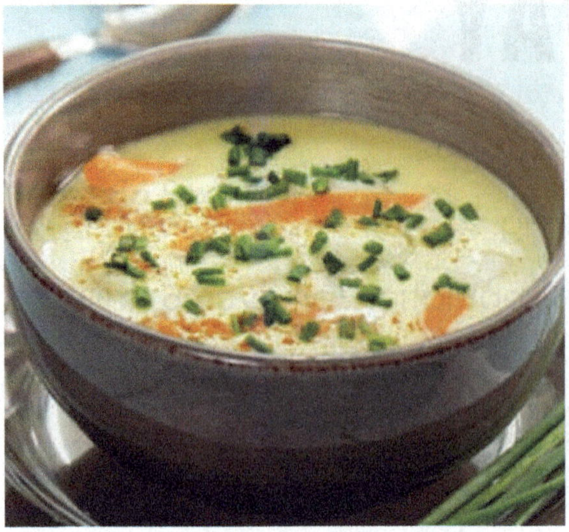

Amount of calories per serving is 416kcal.

INGREDIENTS

For the chive oil

- 1 bunch of chives
- Pinch salt
- 1⁄2 cup olive oil

For the soup

- 1 tbsp. olive oil
- 4 large carrots, diced (1 1/4 cup)
- 2 yellow onions, chopped (2 1/4 cups)
- 2 celery stalks, diced
- 2 tsp. kosher salt, plus more as needed
- 2 cups fish stock
- 1⁄3 cup dry white wine
- 4 cups heavy cream
- 1 cup crème fraîche, or more to taste
- 1 1⁄2 lb. fresh cod, cut into 1-inch cubes
- Bread, for serving (optional)
- Chopped chives, for garnish (optional).

This seafood-lovers soup recipe is a low carb and no-gluten version of the Norwegian fiskesuppe, a one pot delicacy takes about 25 minutes to prepareother fish such as salmon can be used too.

DIRECTIONS

1. To make the chive oil, set a bowl of ice water next to the stove. In a medium saucepan of heavily salted boiling water, add the chives and cook until bright green, about 10 seconds; remove and transfer to the ice water.
2. Squeeze out excess water from the chives, then coarsely chop. Transfer to a blender with a pinch of salt. Slowly stream in the oil, blending on high speed until smooth. Chill, then strain and reserve.
3. To make the soup, in a large pot or Dutch oven, heat the olive oil over medium-high heat. Add the carrots, onion, and celery; season with 1 teaspoon salt and cook, stirring occasionally, for 2 minutes. Add the wine and cook until mostly evaporated, about 6 minutes. Add the stock and bring to a boil; reduce to a simmer and let cook until the vegetables are al dente, 5–8 minutes. Add the cod and cook for 2 minutes. Stir in the cream, crème fraiche, and the remaining 1 teaspoon salt, and bring the soup back to a simmer (for a thicker soup, add more crème fraiche to taste). Taste and adjust the salt as needed.
4. Ladle the soup into bowls. Drizzle with chive oil and serve with bread if desired.

You are likely to find a lot of polar bears in Norway.

CARIBBEAN & CENTRAL AMERICA

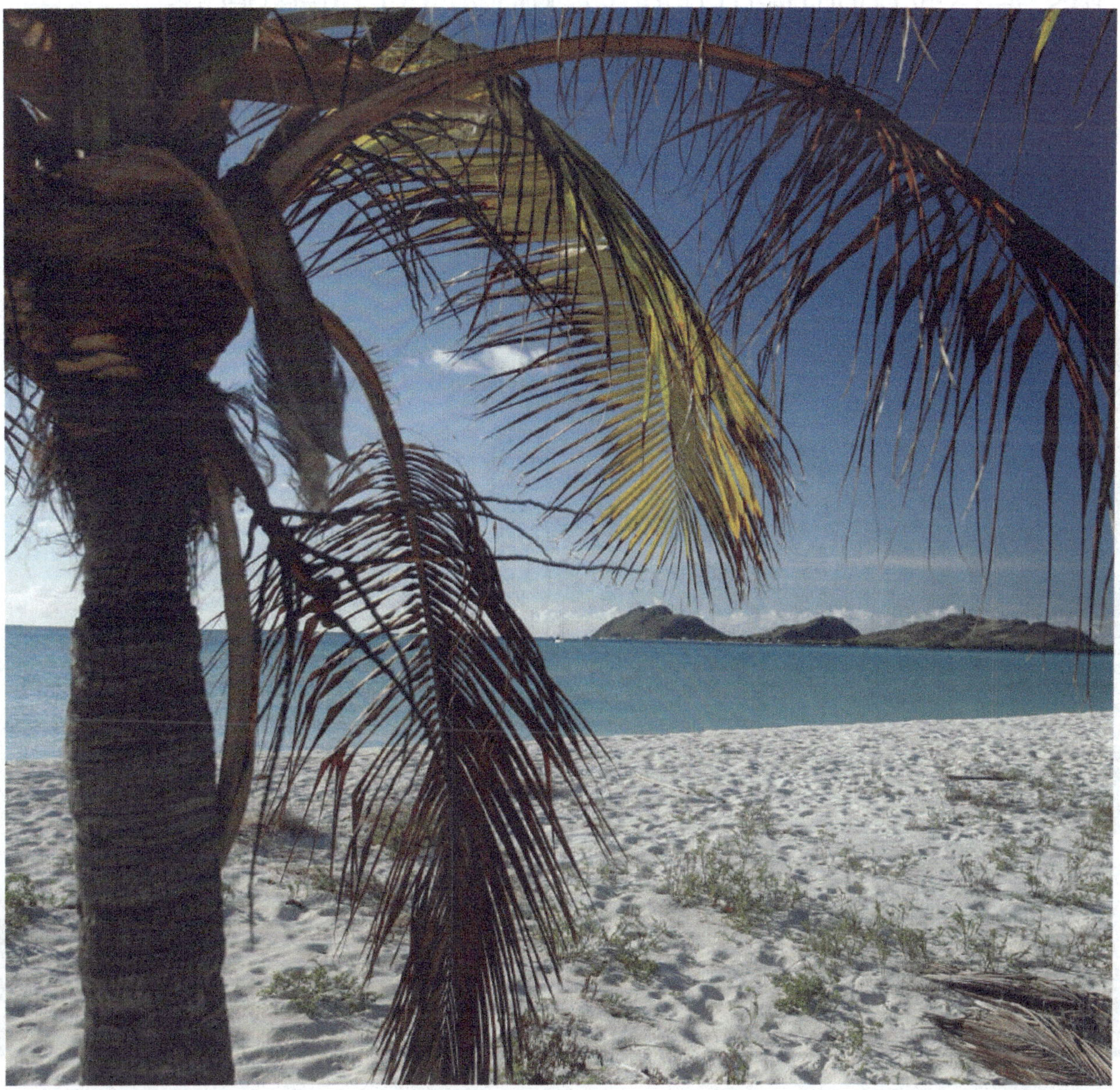

EL SALVADOR

Fondly known as the Land of Volcanoes.

There is only so much you know about El Salvadorans.

Of all the Central American countries, El Salvador is the smallest.

This densely populated country is known for Coffee beans.

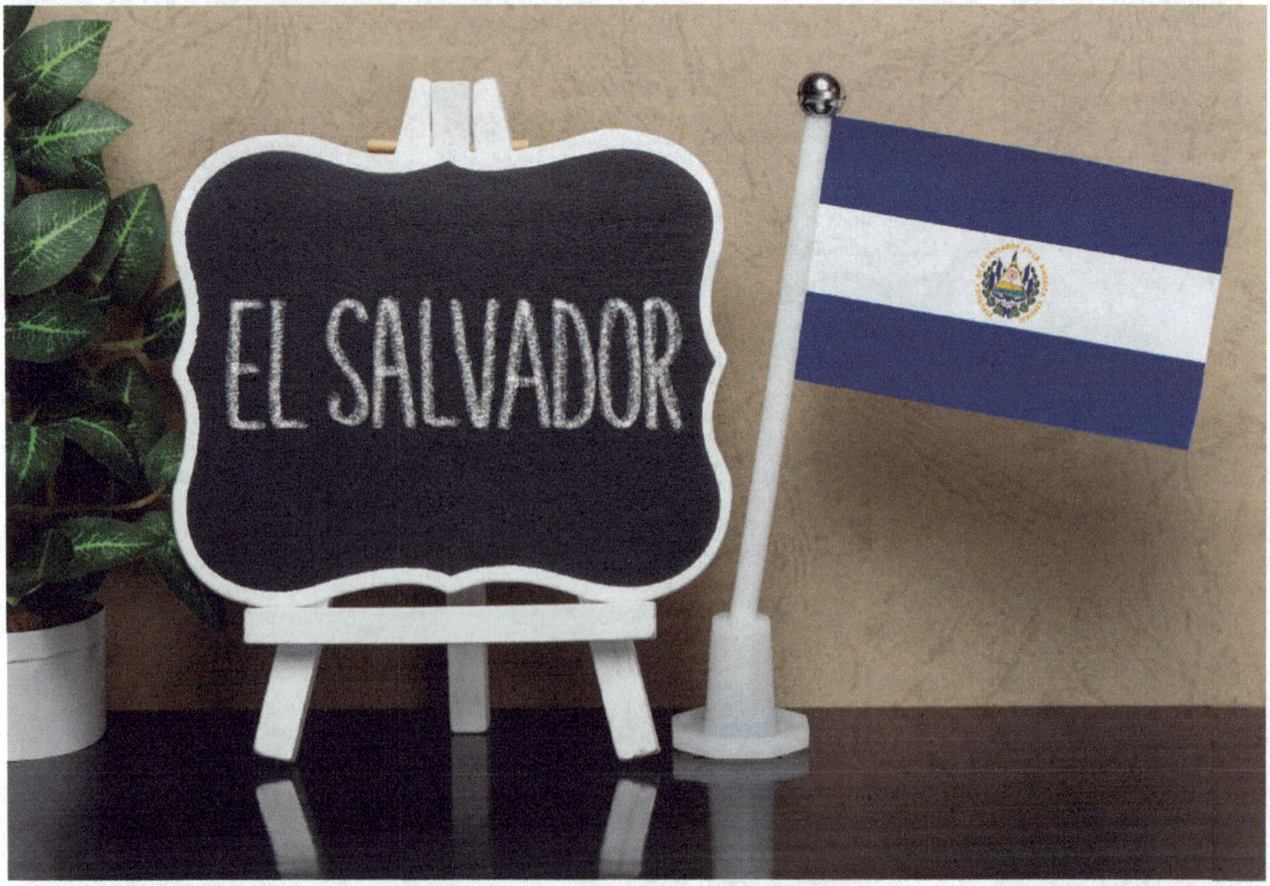

Shrimp Soup (El-Salvador Style)

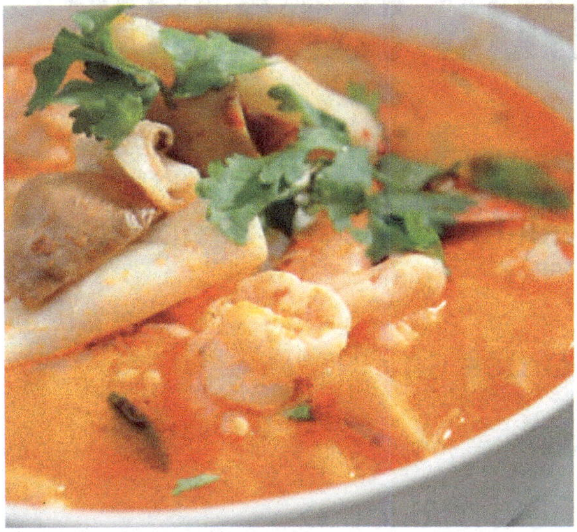

Amount of calories per serving is 273.2

INGREDIENTS

- 4 vegetable oil
- 30 medium shrimp
- 1/2 cup minced onion
- 2 large garlic doves minced
- 1/2 cup chopped cilantro
- 1 cup chopped tomato
- 1/2 cup chopped green bell pepper
- 8 cups water
- 1 tablespoon shrimp or chicken bouillon powder
- 1 teaspoon salt
- 1 cup peeled and cubed potatoes 1-inch cubes
- 1 cup sliced carrots 1/4-inch rounds
- 1/2 cup heavy cream optional

There are many fish and soup recipes to delight yourself in for an experience of El Salvador. For sea-food addicts. It is absolutely inviting.

DIRECTIONS

1. In a deep pot, heat the butter or oil on high until very hot. Add the shrimp, onion, garlic, cilantro, tomato, and green bell pepper, and sauté all these ingredients for about 1 minute.
2. Add and combine the water, bouillon powder, and salt, and bring to a boil. Add the potatoes and carrots, cover, reduce heat to medium, and cook for 10 to 15 minutes or until vegetables are tender.
3. Add the cream, if using, stir, turn the heat off, and remove from stove. Correct the salt, and serve the soup hot, Squeeze the lemon juice on top before eating.

Santa Ana Volcano (Volcánllamatepec) and Lake Coatepeque are two important you must visit for a complete feel of El Salvador.
Exciting possibilities abound in the El Impossible National park!

TURKS AND CAICOS ISLANDS

Turks and Caicos is a British Overseas country.

Clear blue waters, serene resorts, beautiful Islands, and abundant biodiversity are part of this country.

Turks and Ciaos is home to the exotic Grace Bay.

The capital town is called Cockburn Town.

A boat ride across her Islands will not be a bad idea.

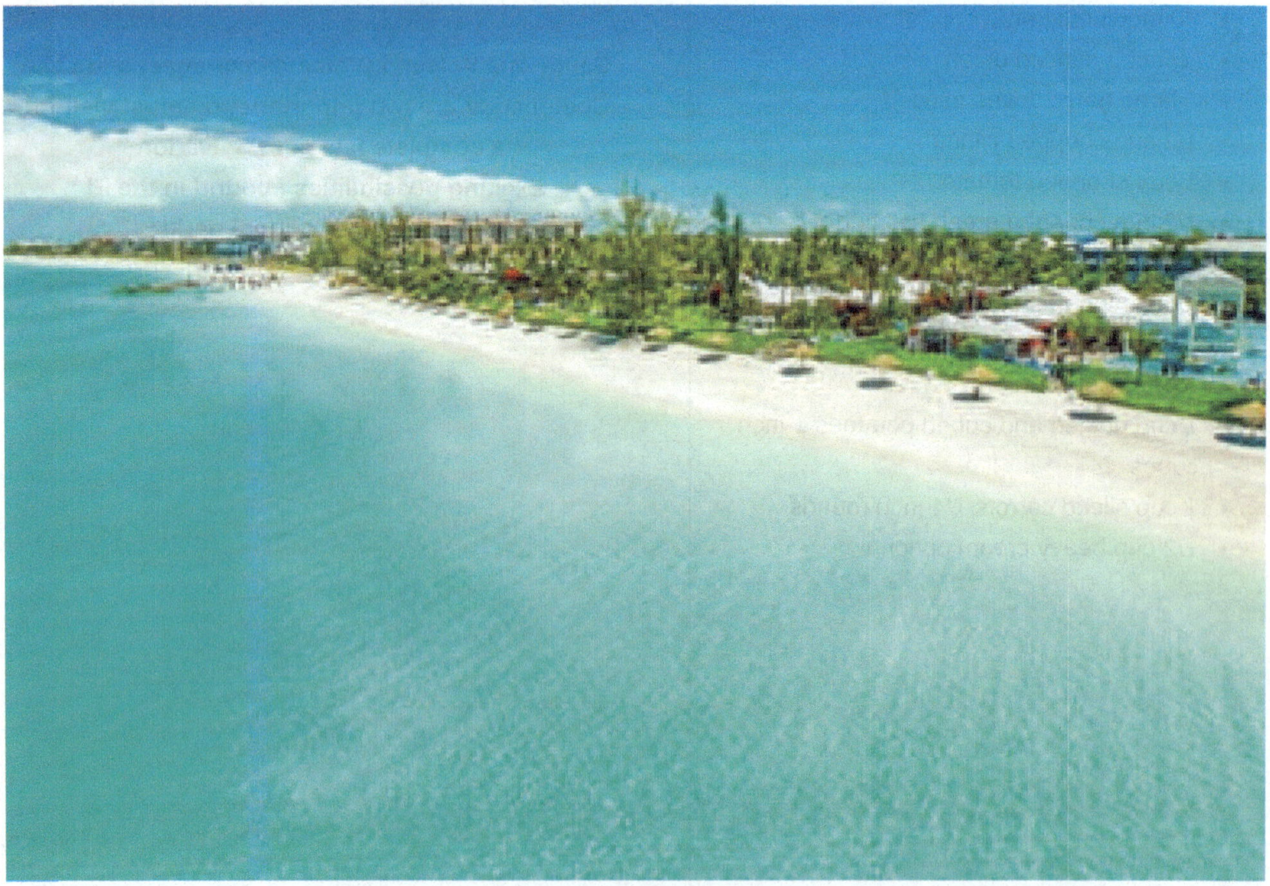

Red Peas Soup

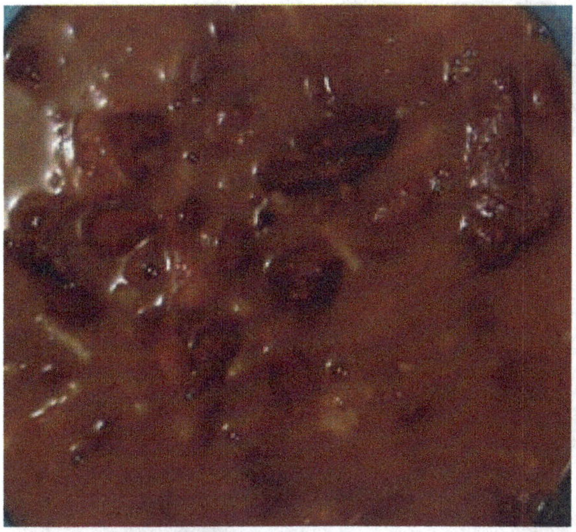

Red Pea Soup is an all-time favorite soup!
It's a thick and flavorful soup with meat, starchy vegetables, and chewy dumplings.
Like most soups, Red Pea Soup is more like a stew. It's the main meal, not a starter soup or one you'd have with salad or a sandwich. Red Pea Soup is very satisfying.

INGREDIENTS

- 1 ½ cups kidney beans, canned or soaked overnight
- 2 pigtails
- 1 carrot, diced
- 1 medium sweet potato(boniato) cut into small cubes
- 8 pimento berries
- ½ medium onion, chopped
- 4 cloves garlic, minced
- 1 scallion, finely chopped
- About 10 sprigs of thyme
- 1 hot pepper, seeded
- 1 tsp black pepper
- 1 ½ tsp salt
- 8 cups water + ¼ cup water
- 1 cup flour

DIRECTIONS

1. To make the soup, boil pigtails in water to remove the salt then repeat the process twice, using fresh water each time.
2. In a large pot add beans, pigtails cut into bite-sized pieces, carrot, sweet potato, pimento, onion, garlic, scallion, thyme, hot pepper, black pepper, and salt, and bring to a boil. Simmer until the peas are tender and a bit mushy.
3. To make spinners place flour, salt, and water in a bowl and mix to form a stiff dough then pinch off small pieces of dough and roll between palms to form an elongated spinner.
4. Add spinners to soup and then cook for an additional 10 minutes

The Iguana Islands is a must-try for animal lovers. Treat yourself to one of the natural drinks on the Islands! It's always worth it.

SOUTH AMERICA

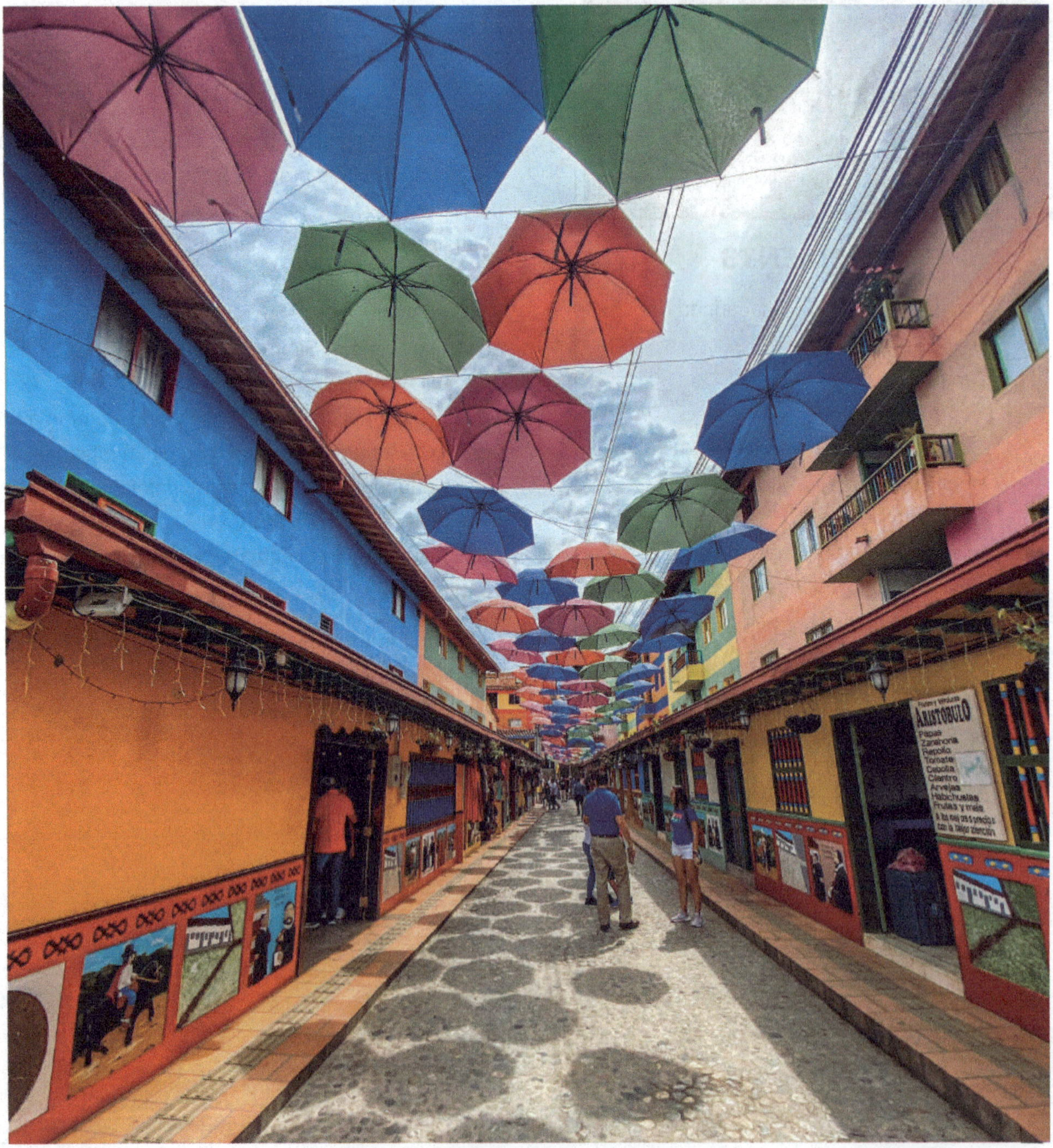

ECUADOR

The capital state of this South American country Quitois famous for certain sacred buildings.

Ecuador boasts of large petroleum reserves, and this accounts for a large portion of its national capital.

Ecuador is a big exporter of coffee, wood, and fish.

It is also renowned for the production of staples like corn, palm and coffee, shrimp, sugar cane, and, rice.

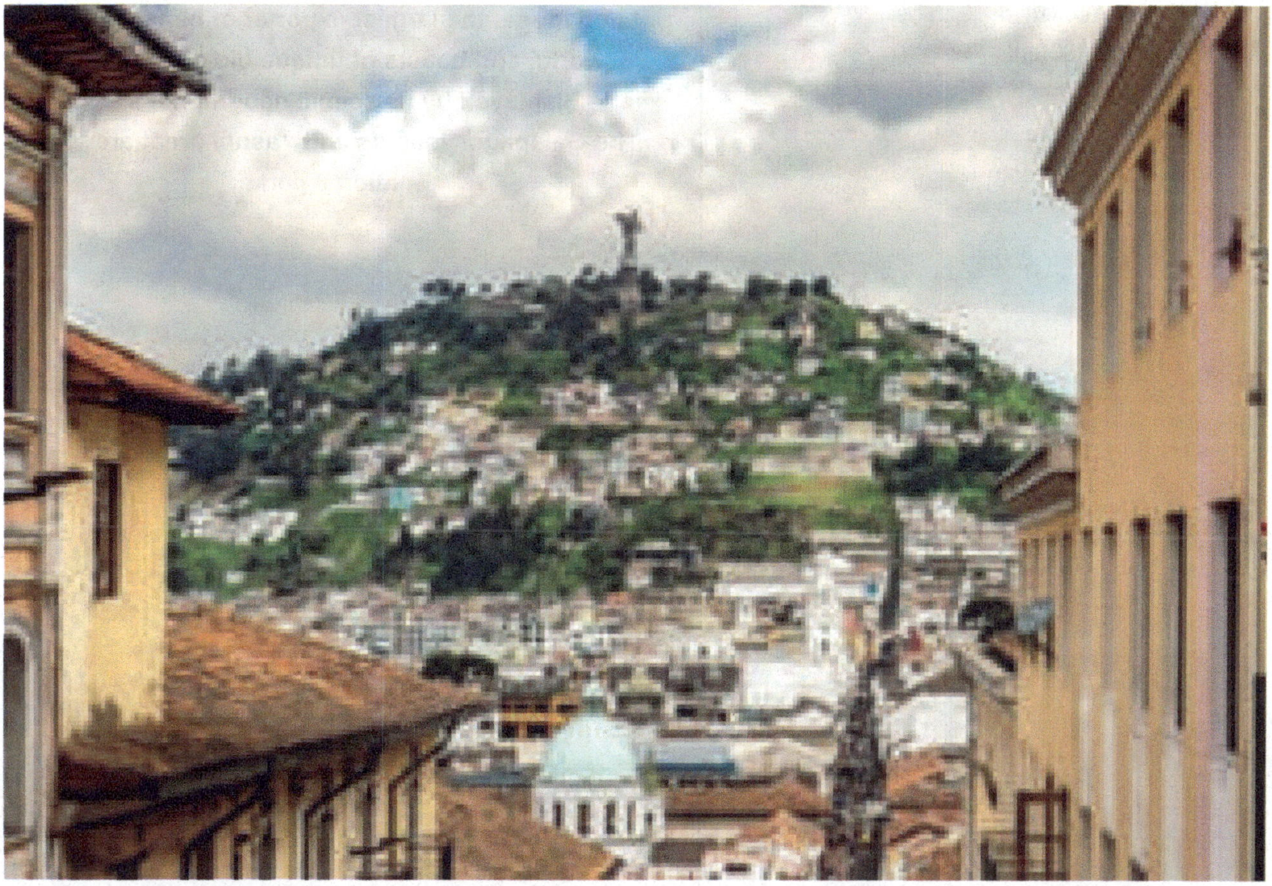

Ecuadorian Carrot Soup

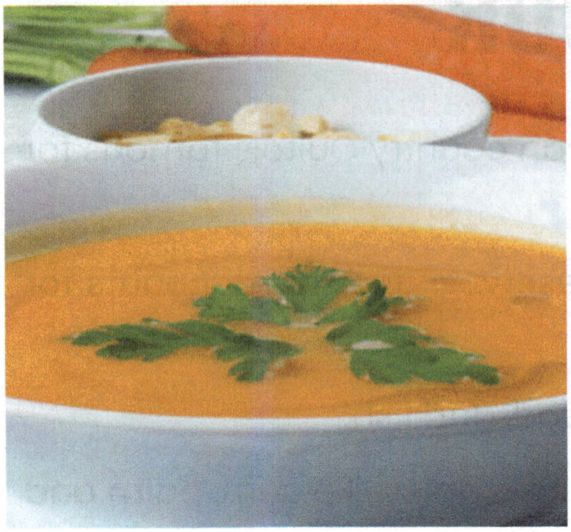

Carrot Soup is also called Potage de Crecy. Typically, a simple carrot soup involves using other root vegetables for extra flavorfor consistency.

You can enjoy the carrot soup served hot or cold – both versions taste delicious.

INGREDIENTS

- Carrots -- 8
- White Onion -- 1
- Water -- 1 liter
- Cream -- 300ml
- Butter -- 5
- Salt -- to taste
- Pepper -- to taste

DIRECTIONS

1. Cut the carrot in six parts and the onion in 4 pieces cook in the water for 30 minutes, blend and strain the preparation, then continue cooking this blended liquid with salt and pepper for 15 minutes more finally add the cream and the butter, then cook 10 minutes more.
2. Don't forget to move with a spoon several times. Serve immediately with optional onion bread on the side.

Ecuador is the largest exporter of bananas in the world, and boasts of unique bio diversities as displayed by its scenic geographic sites:
The Galapagos Islands and Yasuni great arewildlife national parks.

ARGENTINA

The world's eighth-largest country.

The largest city and the capital city is Buenos Aires and borders largely around South America.

Argentina has of a population of over 45,767,250 residents, with major cities as Buenos Aires, Córdoba, Rosario, Mendoza, and Tucumán

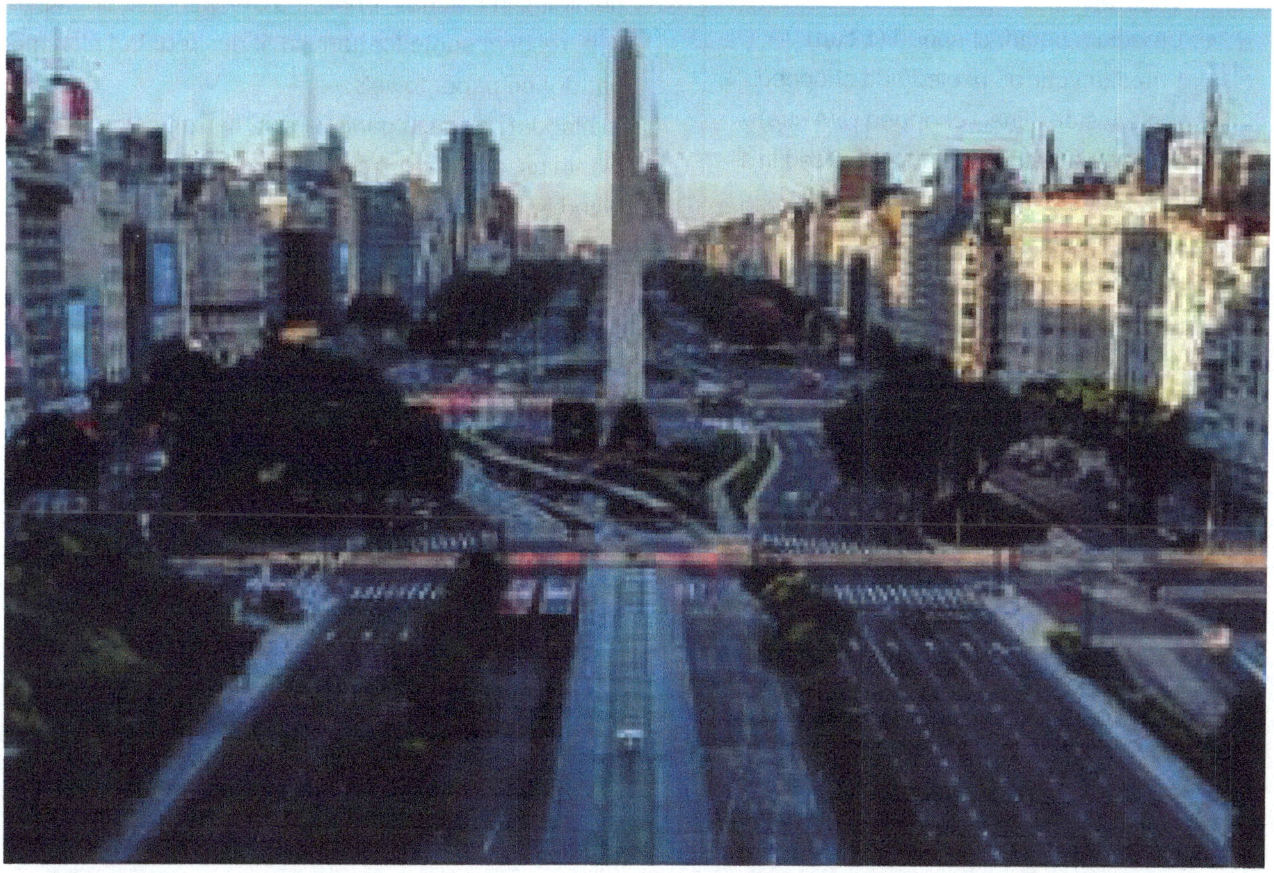

Argentinean Plantain Soup

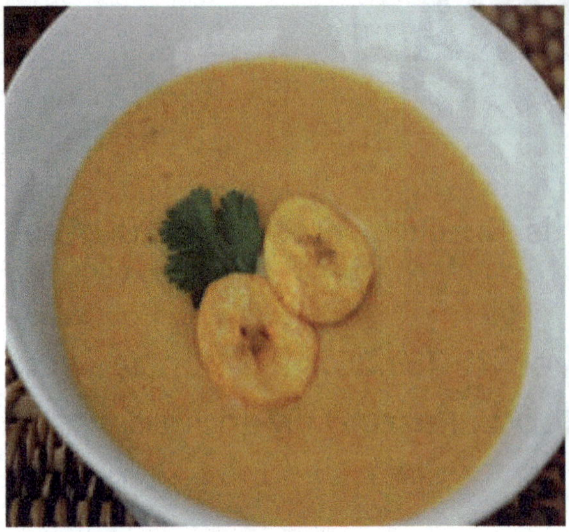

INGREDIENTS

- 3tablespoons olive oil
- 2garlic cloves, peeled and halved lengthwise
- 1 medium onion, chopped (1 cup)
- 1 medium carrot, peeled and chopped
- 1celery stalk, finely chopped (1/4 cup)
- 3green plantains, peeled and sliced in 1-inch slices
- 1cup vegetable oil
- 5 to 7 cups Progresso™ chicken broth (from 2 cartons of 32 oz each)
- 1teaspoon ground cumin
- 1teaspoon salt
- Ground black pepper, if desired
- Cilantro leaves, if desired

Traditional Argentinean soups are based on veggies and rice and the stews also include meat, especially the loved beef.

The traditional plantain soup is quite tasty, with the condition that the plantains are green and not yellow-black.

Looking forward to having dinner in Argentina? You don't want to missArgentinean plantain soup

DIRECTIONS

1. Heat oil in 5-qt Dutch oven over medium heat. Stir in garlic and onions. Cook for 2 to 3 minutes or until onion is transparent. Remove from Dutch oven. Stir in carrot and celery until soft on same Dutch oven. On a separate skillet heat oil over medium heat. Stir in plantains in batches; Fry* for 3 to 5 minutes or until soft, reserve some for garnish, if desired. Let plantains pat-dry on paper towels.
2. In blender, blend in garlic, onion, carrot, celery, plantains, and 4 cups chicken broth (might have to blend in batches). Blend until soft and smooth.
3. Place in same Dutch oven; stir in mixture from blender. Add cumin and salt. Stir in 1 cup of broth or until desired consistency. Serve. If desired, decorate with plantain slices and cilantro leaves.

A taste of Argentina is a taste of palatable food and wine.
Its excellence in performing arts is a sure reason why it tops the charts amongst South American countries.

SECTION 11

LUNCH

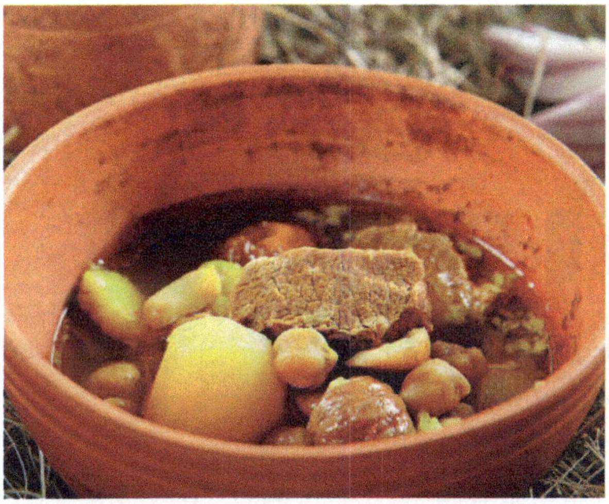
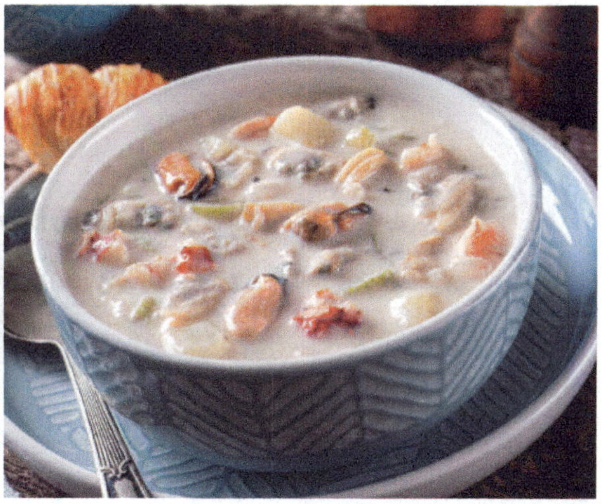
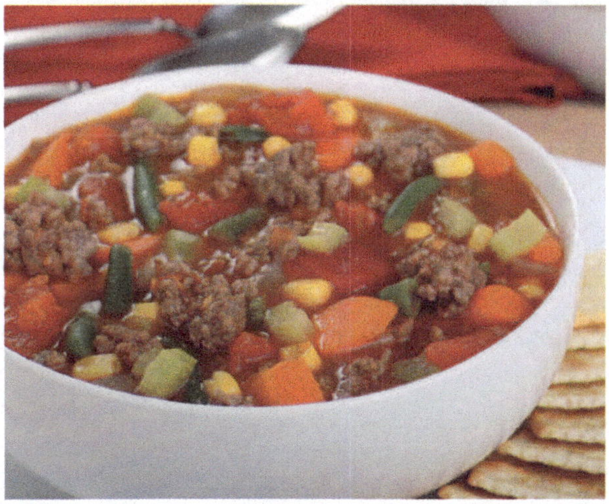
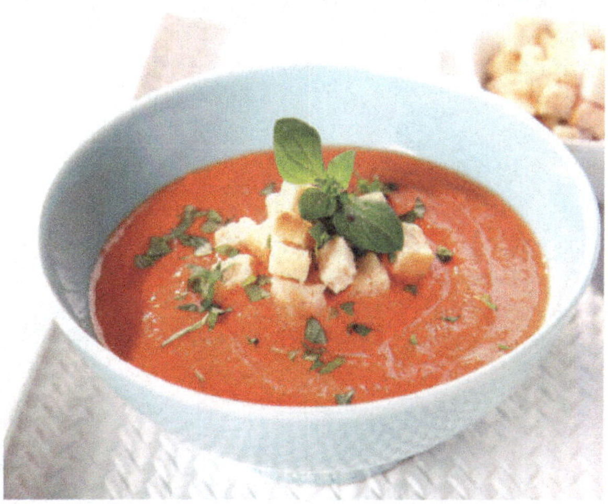

AFRICA

BURUNDI

This country capital city isGitega and the largest city is Bujumbura.

The East African Burundi boasts of rich biodiversity, scenic mountainside, and natural green vegetation.

Lake Tanganyika is a favorite tourist spot for nature lovers.

Food like potatoes, maize, and rice are cultivated and form a major part of Burundi staple diets

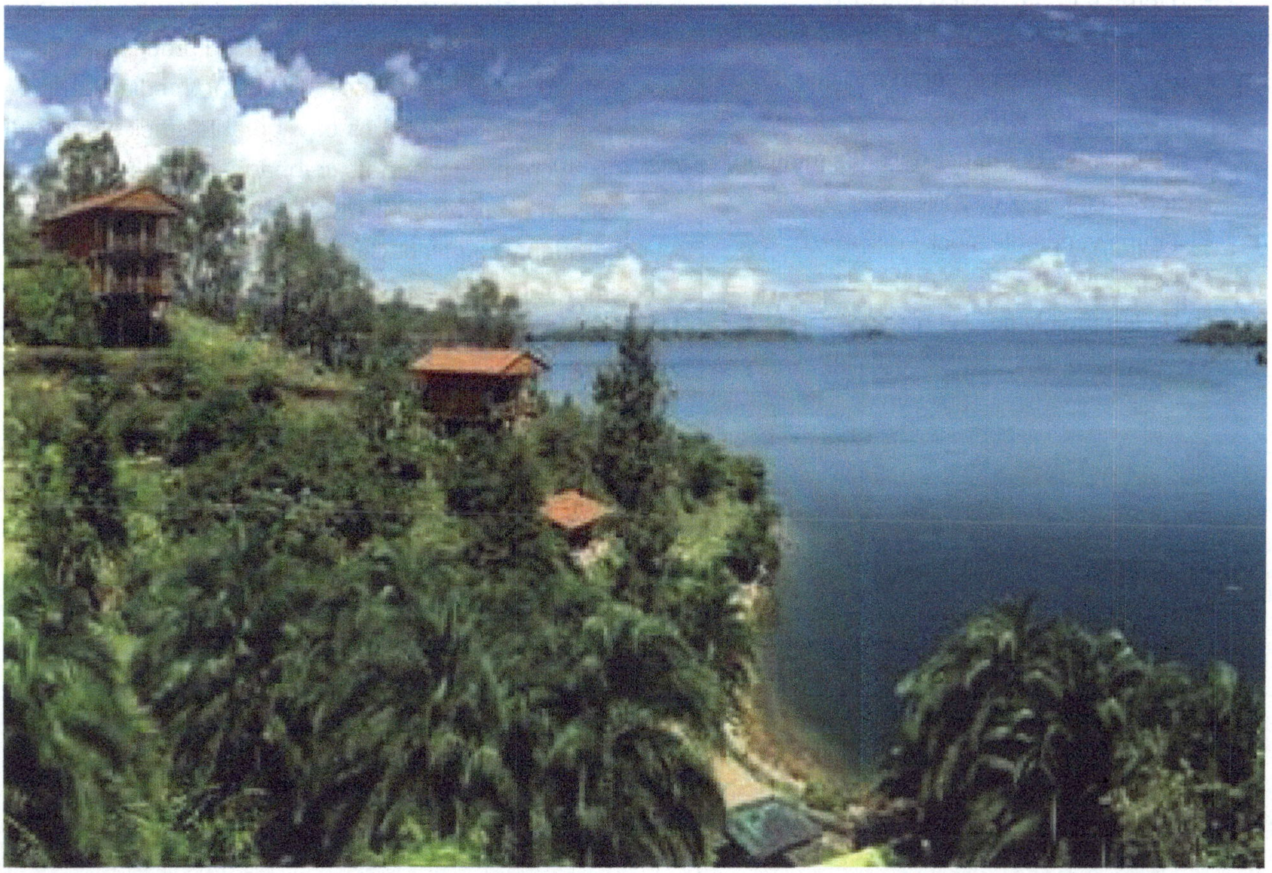

Burundian Lentil and Bean Soup

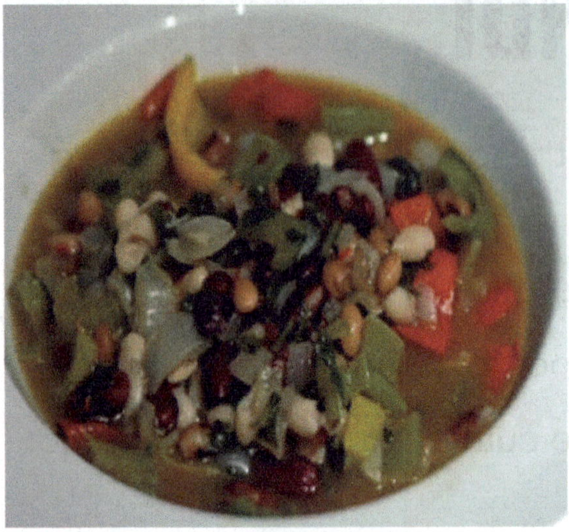

Lentil and bean soup is a super delicious and protein-rich soup with great healthy benefits. It is filled with sweet veggies and will warm you up during the cold.

INGREDIENTS

- 1 large sweet potato, peeled and cut into small cubes
- 3 large carrots, peeled and diced
- 2 small yellow onions, peeled and diced
- 1/2 green cabbage, cored and shredded
- 1 1/2 cup brown lentils
- 1/2 lb. fresh green beans, ends trimmed and cut into 1-2 inch pieces
- 4 cups vegetable stock
- 1/2 tsp salt
- 1/4 tsp freshly ground black pepper
- 2 tbs olive oil

DIRECTIONS

1. Place a large soup pot over medium heat. Once the pot is hot, add the olive oil. When the olive oil starts to simmer, add the diced onions and cook, stirring occasionally, for 5 minutes.
2. Once the onions are soft and the edges are starting to brown, add the lentils and cook for 1 minutes, stirring constantly to ensure that the lentils are evenly coated in the hot oil.
3. Add 2 1/2 cups of vegetable stock to the lentils, stir a few times, lower the heat to medium-low, cover, bring the pot to a simmer, and cook for 20 minutes. Stir the lentils a few times during the cooking process.
4. After 20 minutes, increase the heat to medium, add the remaining 1 1/2 cups of vegetable stock along with the sweet potato, carrots, cabbage, and green beans. Season everything with the salt and pepper and stir to thoroughly combine. Cover and bring the pot to a simmer. Once the stock is simmering, cook for 20 more minutes, stirring every 5 minutes or so.
5. After the second 20 minutes, check to see if the lentils are starting to burst and turn to mush. If so, the dish is ready. If you want this to be more of a soup and less of a thick stew, add more vegetable stock to your liking. Otherwise, spoon the thick vegetable dish into bowls and serve hot!

Embrace the true African culture in Bujumbura! Do not forget to sample the delights of the Rusizi River National Park.

LIBYA

The North African countryis officially called the State of Libya.

The population of Libya is estimated at 7,022,065 and its capital is Tripoli.

The arid lands, stocked with oil reserves in abundance.

The El Kouf National Park is known for its hilly paths, water-embedded lands and natural serenity.

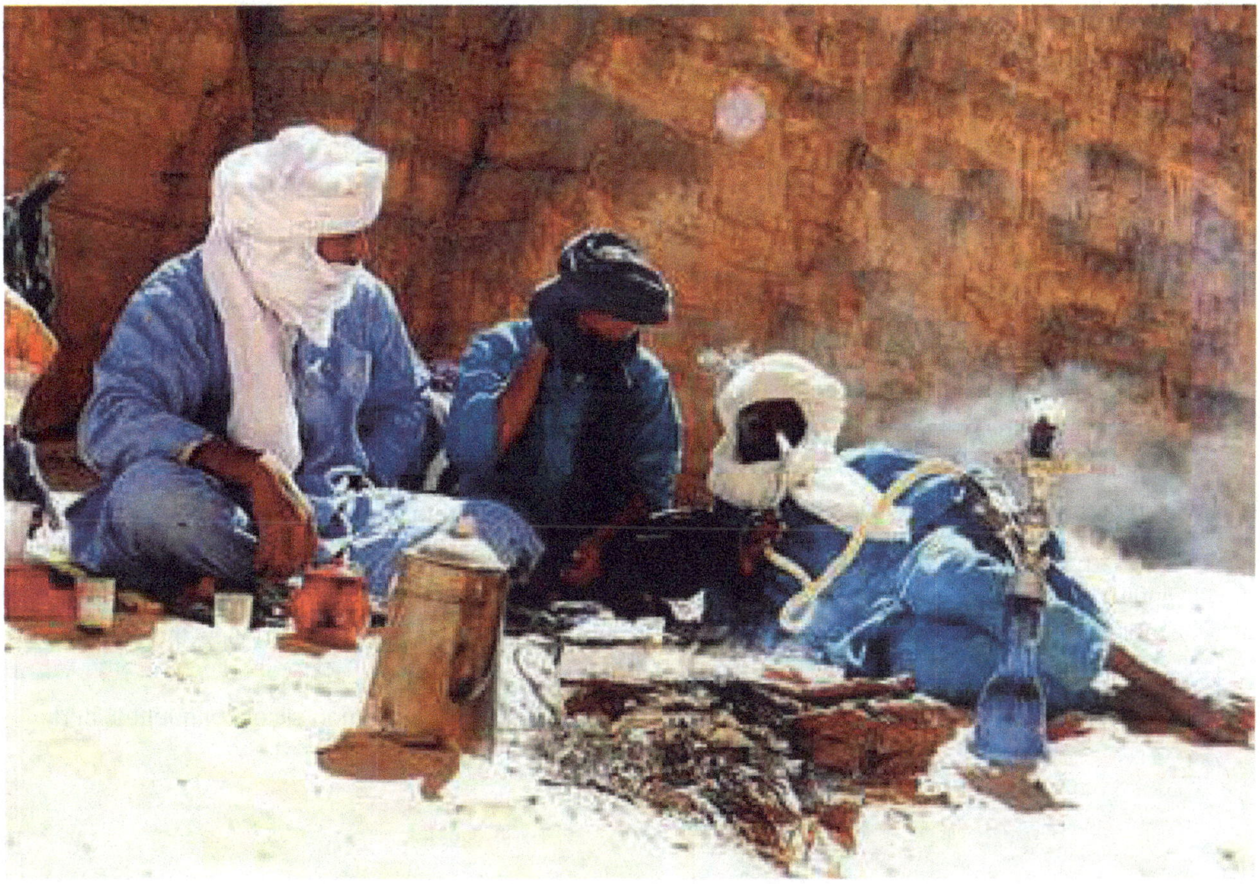

Libyan Lamb Soup - Libyan Sharba

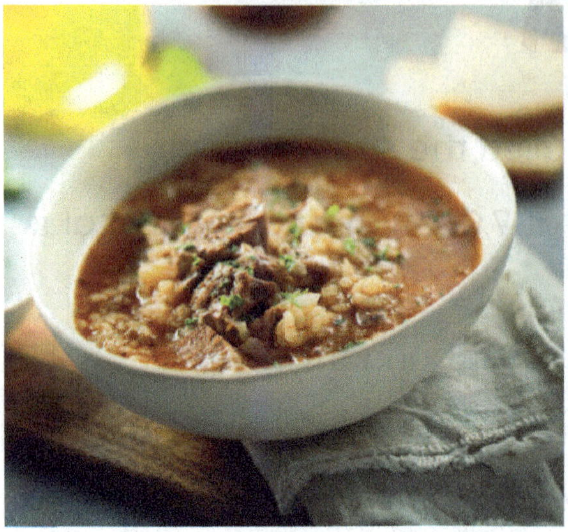

Amount of calories per serving is 267.

INGREDIENTS

- 1 tablespoon olive oil
- 1 medium onion, diced
- 200g lamb meat, boneless, diced into small cubes
- 1 teaspoon harissa
- 1 teaspoon turmeric
- 1 teaspoon sea salt
- 1/2 teaspoon ground pepper, freshly ground
- 1/4 teaspoon cayenne or paprika
- 2 heaping tablespoons of tomato paste
- 1 14oz can of chickpeas
- 1/3 cup of orzo pasta
- 1 tsp ground caraway or Libyan baharat*
- 1/4 cup fresh herbs; parsley, dill, or cilantro
- 2 tablespoons dried mint

The Libyan Lamb soup is a simple and tasty soup that's sure to be a welcome guest on your table. This is a tomato-based soup, with warming North African spices, lamb, chickpeas, and orzo pasta. It's a delicious one-pot meal.

DIRECTIONS

1. Heat oil in a 3qts pot at medium-high heat. Add onions and saute until golden.
2. Once onions are golden, add turmeric, cayenne, harissa paste, salt and pepper. Give everything a good stir. Then add tomato paste and continue cooking for 1-2 minutes - At this point, the oil should turn red. That's the look we're going for here.
3. Now stir in your lamb and ensure all of the spice mixture coats the meat. Lower the heat to low. You're looking for a soft simmer the fat from the lamb will create liquid; don't add water yet. Just cover and forget about it for 5-7 minutes.
4. After the meat has released its juices remove the lid and add 1 1/2 cups and bring to a rapid boil. Once the rapid boil has been achieved, reduce heat to a gentle simmer for 10 minutes.
5. Add in your cooked chickpeas along with 2 1/2 cups of hot water—Cook for 15 minutes.
6. Add in orzo pasta, garlic and caraway. cook for 5 -7 minutes. Once the pasta is cooked add the parsley or your fresh herb of choice.
7. The last set to making this soup is the mint! Take 1 tablespoon of the dried mint place it in your hands and rub your hand together over the soup. They should fall into the soup as a fine powder. Allow the mint to cook for a few minutes.
8. Serve the soup with lemon slices, baguettes, and salad.

ASIA

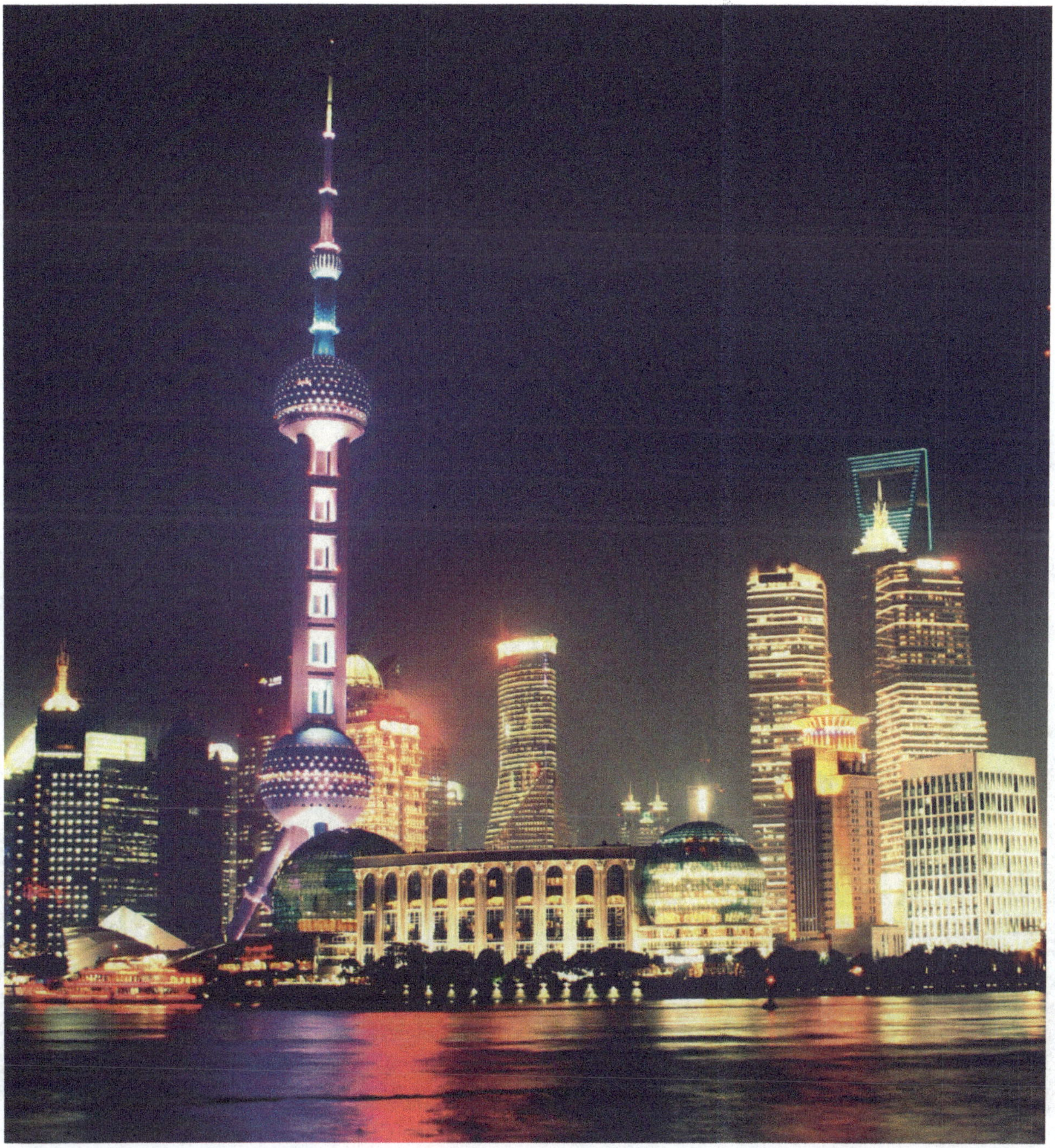

JORDAN

Jordan is an Arabic country nation.

Ever wanted to see the pre-historic archaeology of Petra?

You need to visit Petra city.

It is an arid environment and home to one of the oldest civilizations around the world.

The capital city of Jordan is called Amman.

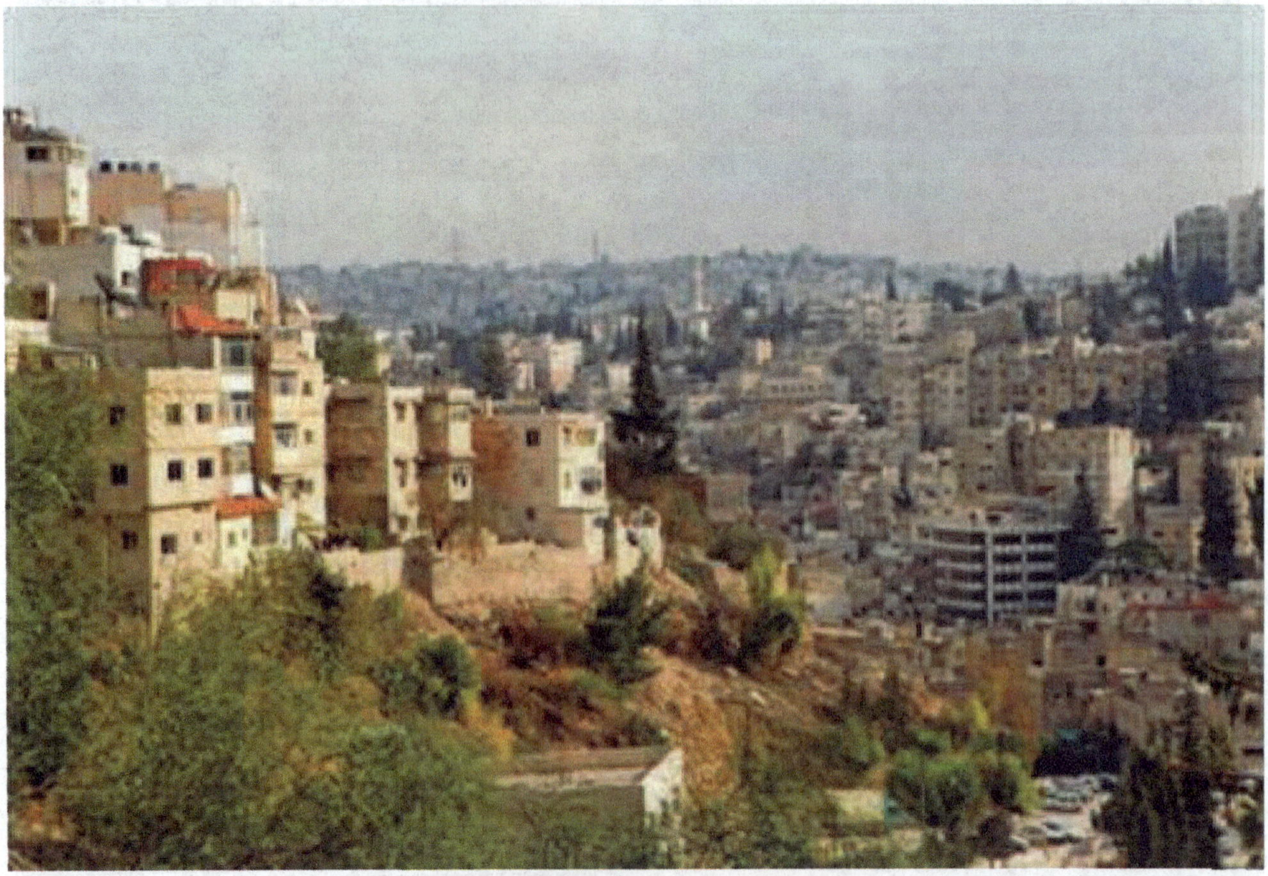

Jordanian Tomato Soup

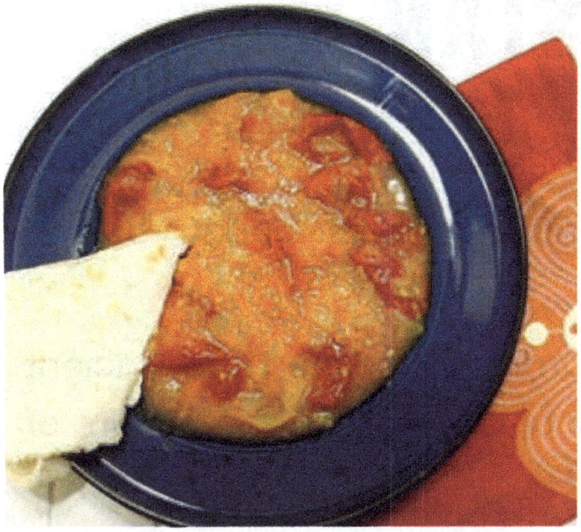

Amount of calories per serving is 49.2

INGREDIENTS

- 1/4 cup butter
- 1 onion chopped
- 2 tomatoes chopped (or 10 cocktail tomatoes)
- 1 teaspoon tomato paste
- 1 cinnamon stick
- pinch of black pepper
- 1 teaspoon salt
- 4 cups water

This Jordanian Tomato Soup gives a lovely buttery and slightly sweet taste with the exotic touch of cinnamon.
Serve with rice or bread as the Jordanians prefer.

DIRECTIONS

1. Melt the butter and fry in it the onions over medium heat until tender in a medium saucepan.
2. Add tomatoes, paste, black pepper, cinnamon stick, salt and water. Bring to a boil, reduce heat and simmer for 60 minutes. Add water if necessary.
3. Serve with a flat bread or rice.

KAZAKHSTAN

The South Asian country with a population of 19,139,158.

Its capital is Nur-Sultan. Kazakhstan is the richest country in the region of South Asia.

A visit to Bayterek tower views &AkOrda Palace and the ancient rocks in the capital city are not optional to embrace the culture of this country.

Lovers of aviary will absolutely love the Saryarka plains!

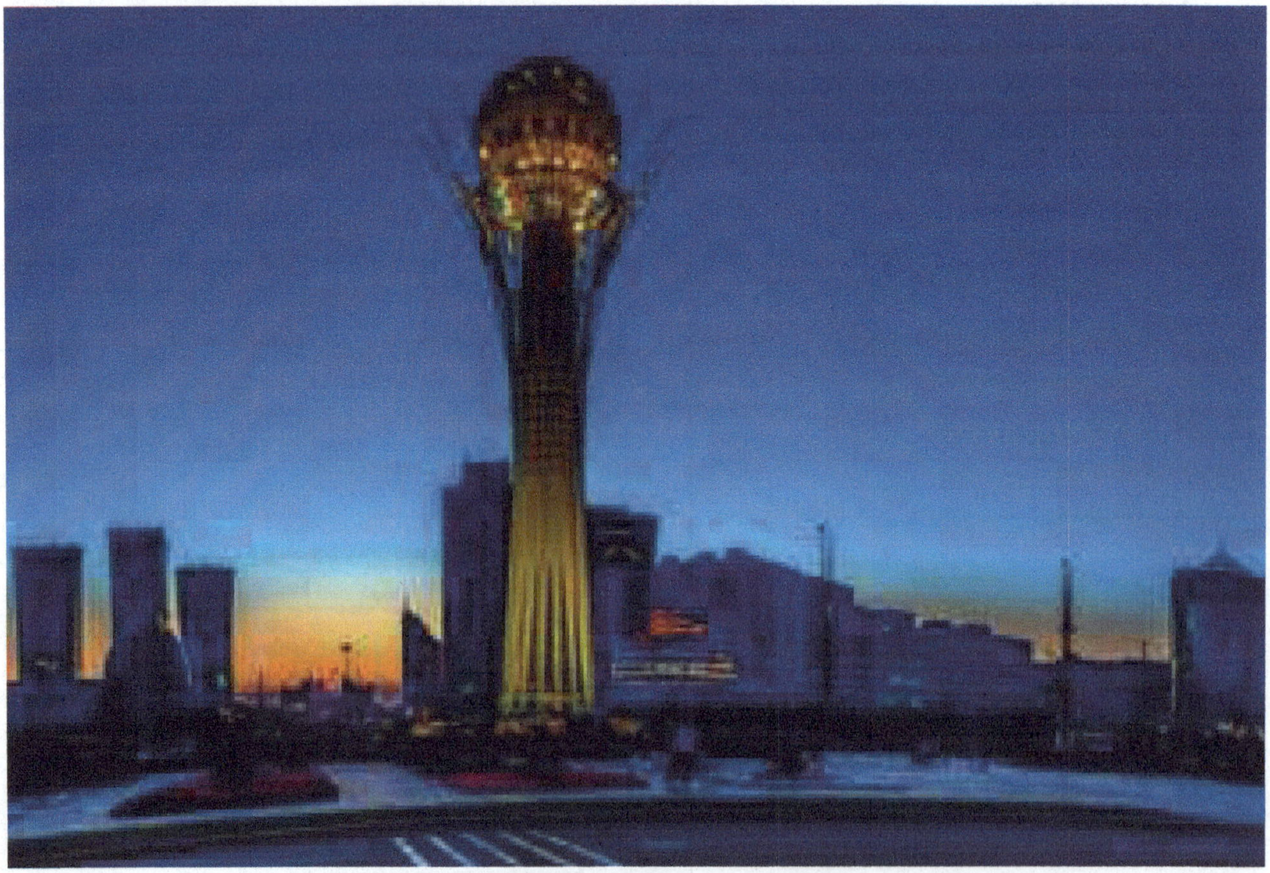

Kazakh Beef Soup

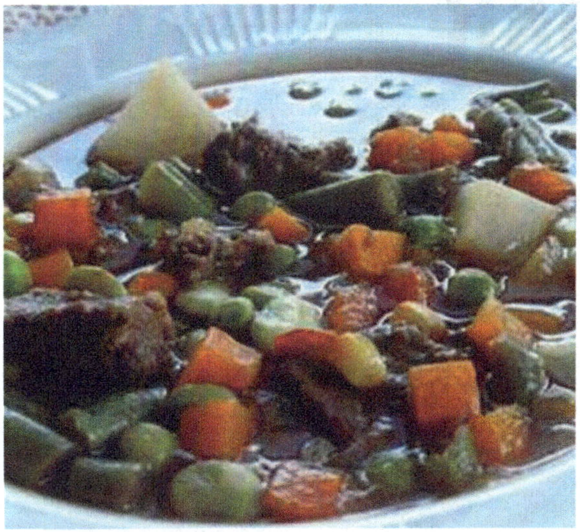

Amount of calories per serving is 49.2

INGREDIENTS

- 3 beef soup bones
- 2 tablespoons olive oil, divided
- 1 (16 ounce) jar sauerkraut - rinsed and drained
- 1 onion, chopped
- 2 large baking potatoes, peeled and cubed
- 1 tablespoon hot chili sauce, or to taste
- salt to taste
- 1/4 cup sour cream (optional)

The word 'kavardak' in Russian means 'shambles' or 'mess', which is where this meal gets its name from.
It's a mess of meat, potatoes, onions, and carrots, all mixed up. Some people add tomatoes and red peppers. You really could throw anything into it. Kavardak Beef Stew is also known as Kaurdak, Kuurdak, Kuyrdak and Kavurdak.

DIRECTIONS

1. Place soup bones in a stock pot with enough water to cover them by 2 inches. Bring to a boil, and cook uncovered for about 1 hour to make beef stock. Remove bones, and cool.
2. Heat one tablespoon of oil in a large skillet. Sauté sauerkraut for a few minutes, then add just enough water to cover the sauerkraut, cover the pan, and let simmer over low heat for about 30 minutes, until the sour taste is gone. Drain, and set aside. Heat remaining olive oil in a small skillet over medium-high heat. Sauté onion in the hot oil until tender.
3. When the bones are out of the stock, add potatoes, and boil for about 15 minutes, until potatoes are tender. Stir in the sauerkraut, onions, and any meat that can be picked from the bones. Season with chili sauce and salt to taste. Simmer over low heat for about 15 minutes. Ladle into bowls, and serve with a dollop of sour cream.

A taste of chilled bozo is a taste of (a foamy drink made from processed grain).

MYANMAR

Myanmar is a multi-ethnic Southeast Asian country.

Its capital is Naypyidaw.

It was formerly called Burma.

Cycling on the roads of Mandalay is a favorite sport for visitors to Myanmar.

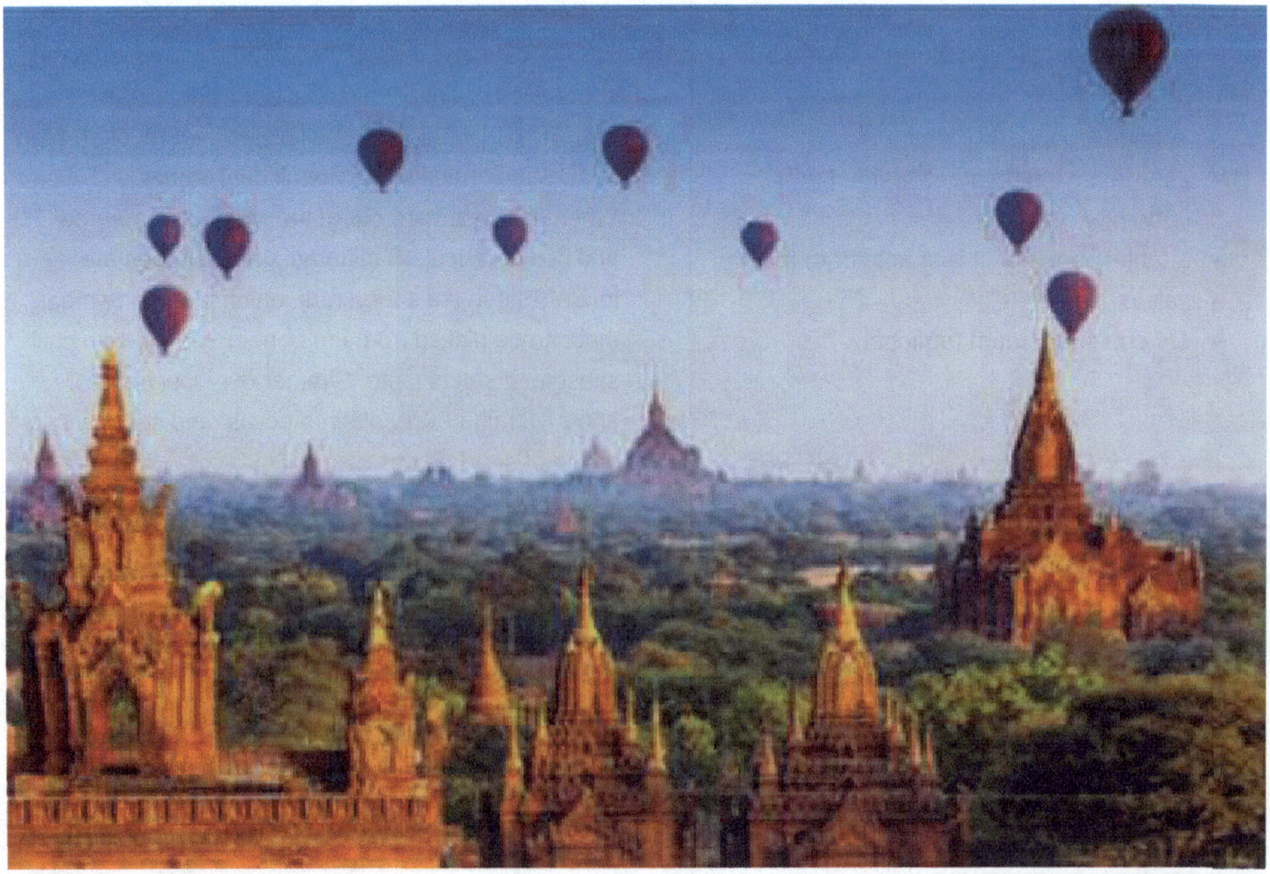

Mohinga (Burmese Fish Soup)

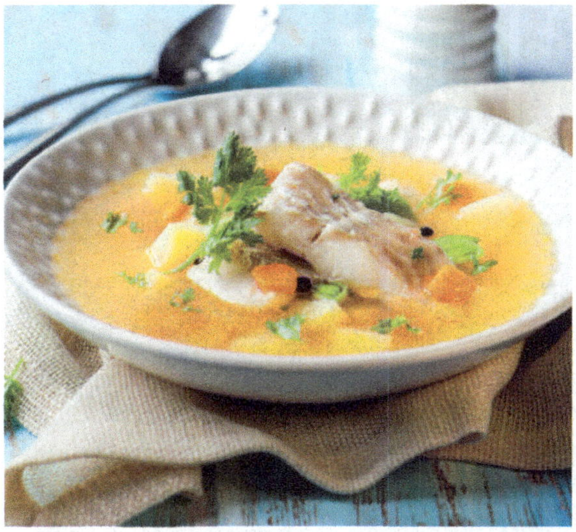

Amount of calories per serving is 588kcal.

For some nations, the national dish offers nothing more than hollow symbolism for the cuisine.
For others, however, the national dish holds a far greater significance and lends a far deeper meaning to the overall national identity.
The country of Myanmar (formerly Burma) falls into this latter category.
For a once proud nation ransacked by intergroup conflicts and civil war, just about anything that brings popular common consensus is a welcome reprieve.
The delightful dish of mohinga is one such reprieve

INGREDIENTS

- 1 tbsp gram (chickpea) flour
- 2 tbsp ground rice or rice flour
- 2 lemongrass stalks, trimmed and finely chopped
- 2 whole dried red chilies, finely chopped, or 2 tspchili flakes
- 1 large onion, finely chopped
- 4 garlic cloves, crushed
- 2.5cm piece fresh ginger, grated
- 4 tbsp groundnut or vegetable oil
- 1 tsp ground turmeric
- 1 tsp ground paprika
- 2 x 110g tins mackerel fillets in brine (undrained)
- 4 tbsp fish sauce, plus extra to serve
- 8 small shallots, peeled
- 400g rice vermicelli noodles
- To serve...
- 100g fresh coriander, chopped
- 3 duck eggs or 6 hen's eggs, hard-boiled and sliced or halved
- 1 red onion, finely sliced
- 3 limes, cut into wedges
- Ready-made deep-fried crispy onions for sprinkling (check these are gluten free, if they need to be)
- Chili flakes to taste
- Large pestle and mortar or mini food processor

DIRECTIONS

1. Toast the gram flour over a low heat in a dry frying pan, stirring often, until it turns golden – keep watch of it so it doesn't burn. Set aside, then toast the ground rice or rice flour in the same way.
2. In a large pestle and mortar, pound the lemongrass, chilies, onion, garlic and ginger to a paste (or use a mini food processor).
3. Heat the oil in a large deep saucepan over a medium heat. Add the turmeric, paprika and the lemongrass/chili paste, then fry for 5-7 minutes until the onion in the paste starts to caramelize.
4. Stir in the mackerel (with the brine), then cook for 5 minutes more, ensuring all the mackerel is coated with the paste.
5. Add the toasted gram and rice flours and keep stirring until the paste thickens.
6. Pour in 1.5 liters water and add the fish sauce. Bring the soup up to the boil, then reduce the heat and simmer for 15 minutes.
7. Add the whole shallots and a pinch of pepper to the soup, thensimmer gently for 30 minutes more (see Make Ahead).
8. Meanwhile, put the vermicelli in a separate large heatproof bowl and pour over boiling water from the kettle. Leave to soak for 7 minutes (or until the noodles are soft), then drain.
9. To serve, divide the vermicelli noodles among 6 bowls. Ladle over the fish soup (leaving behind the whole shallots), then garnish with coriander, halved eggs, red onion, fresh lime wedges, extra fish sauce, crispy onions and chilli flakes.

OCEANIA

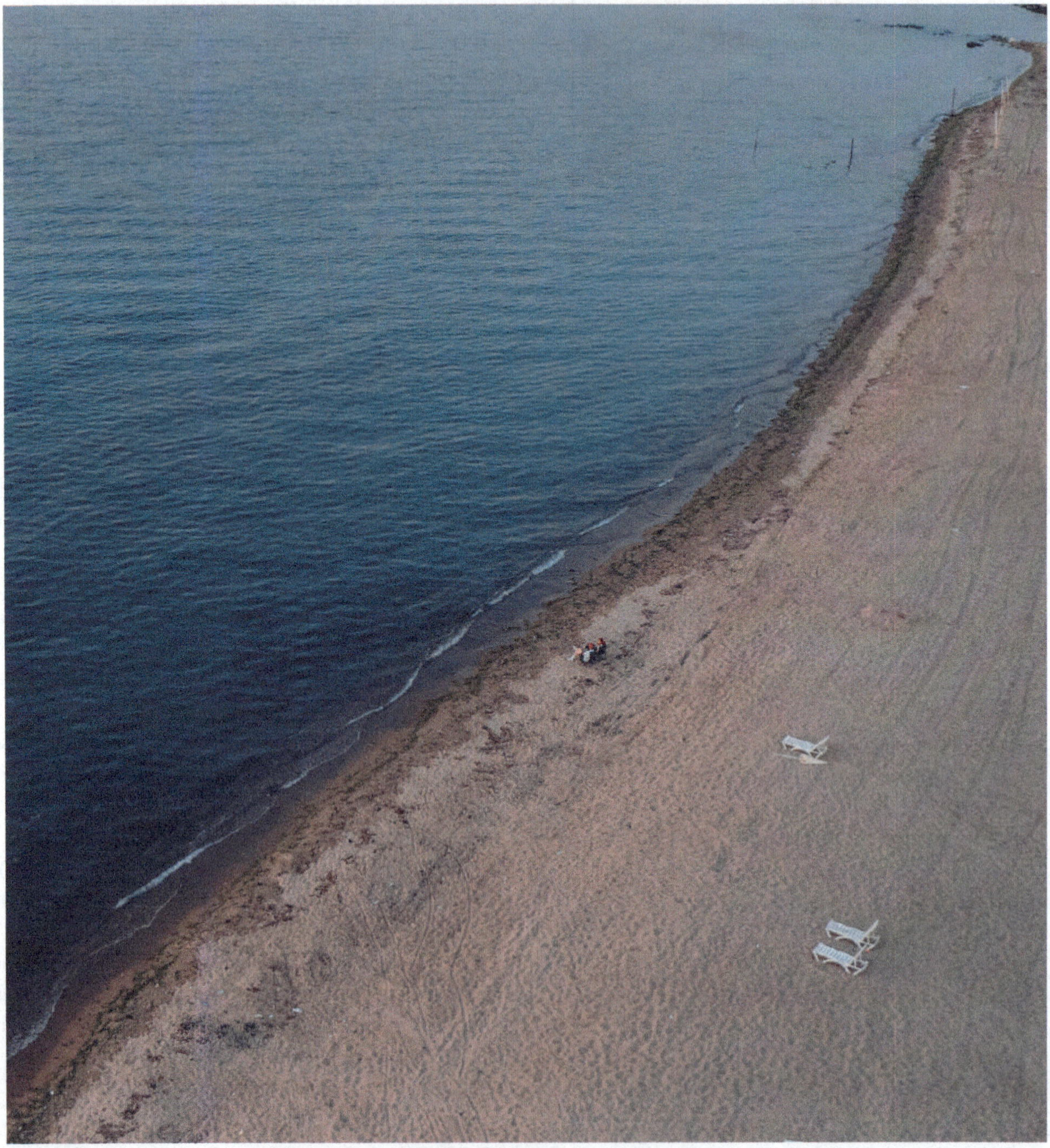

GUAM

Guam is a region in the West Pacific located around the Southeast Asian region.

It is an Island, and its state Capital is Hagatna.

This southern island covers the largest in the Mariana Islands.

Pristine beaches and transparent water bodies are just a bit of Guam.

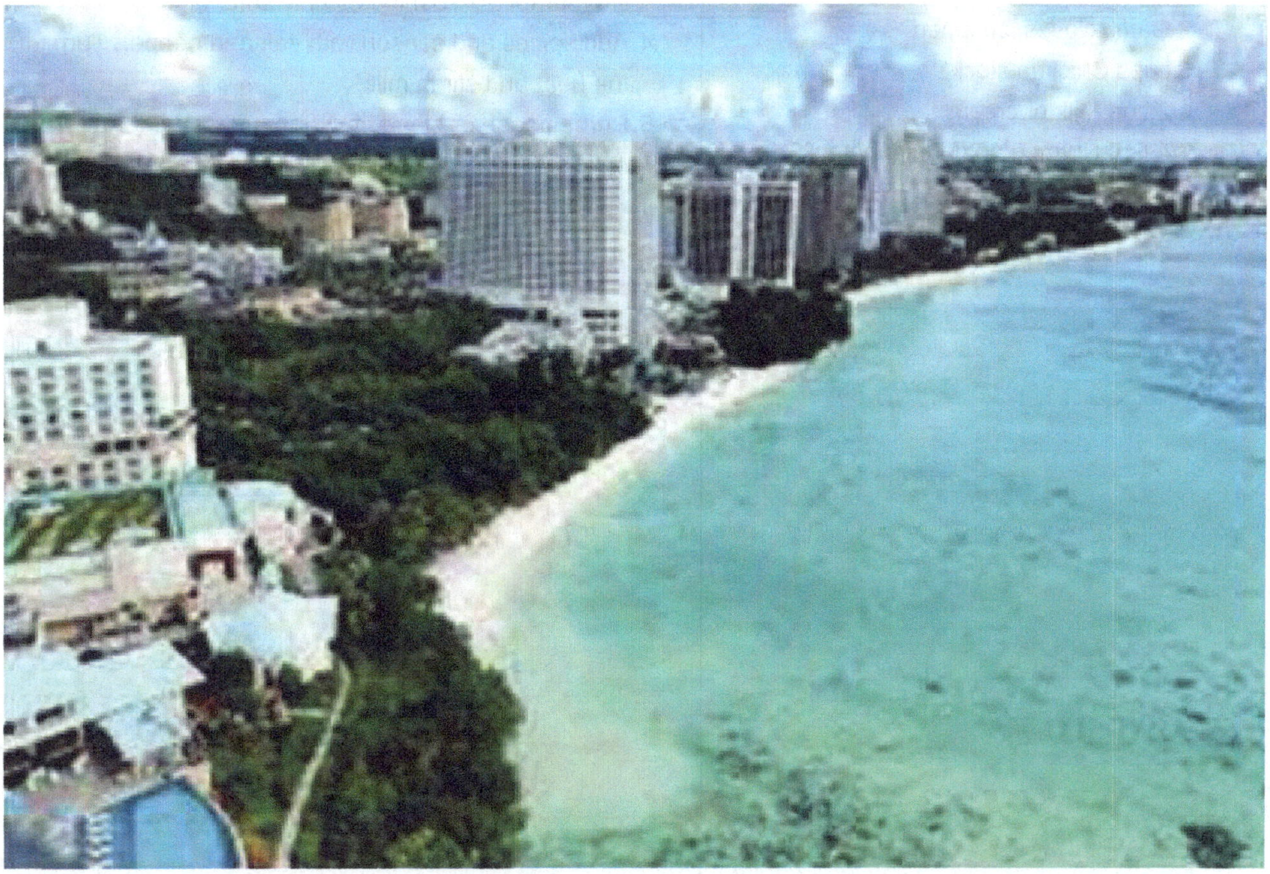

Kabocha Soup

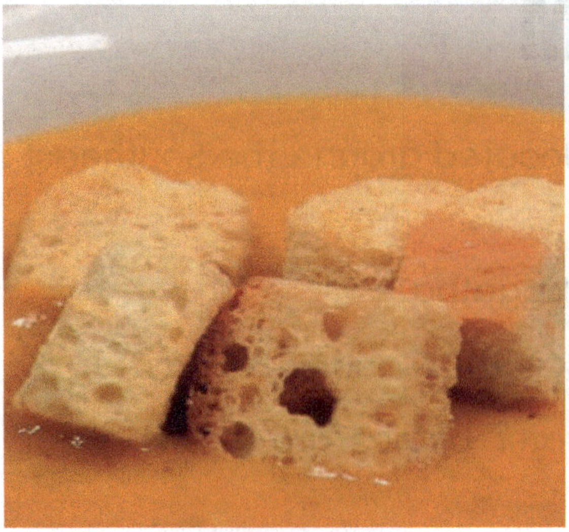

INGREDIENTS

- 3 lbs. Kabocha squash, with or without skin
- 1/4 cup Onion, chopped
- 2 Garlic cloves, chopped
- 6 cups Chicken stock*
- 1/2 cup Milk or cream*
- 1/4 tsp. Nutmeg and/or cinnamon*
- Salt & pepper to taste

Kabocha Soup, which is also known as Kabocha is a thick creamy soup that's made from Kabocha squash, aromatics, and stock.
Instant varieties are available all year round, and in fall, there are pumpkin soup-flavored snack foods like potato chips and instant noodles.
Although it's pretty like a Western winter squash soup, the main difference is that Kabocha Squash Soup is often eaten for breakfast.

DIRECTIONS

1. Kabocha prep: You can roast or steam quartered kabocha for easier peeling or cutting.
2. Cut kabocha into 1" wedges.
3. Sauté onion and garlic until translucent. Add kabocha to the pot and cover with stock. Boil and reduce to a simmer for 10-15 minutes until soft.
4. Add spices and season with salt and pepper. Turn off the heat and stir in milk.
5. Puree, mash or blend the soup and serve for a delicious taste of autumn.

SOLOMON ISLAND

The country in Oceania with a conglomerate of about six major islands and other smaller islands in the South Pacific.

The state capital is Honiara.

This country is uniquely identified for its biodiversity in flora and fauna.

The richness in diversity of many plant and animal species makes Solomon Island a standout amongst many bio-diverse nations.

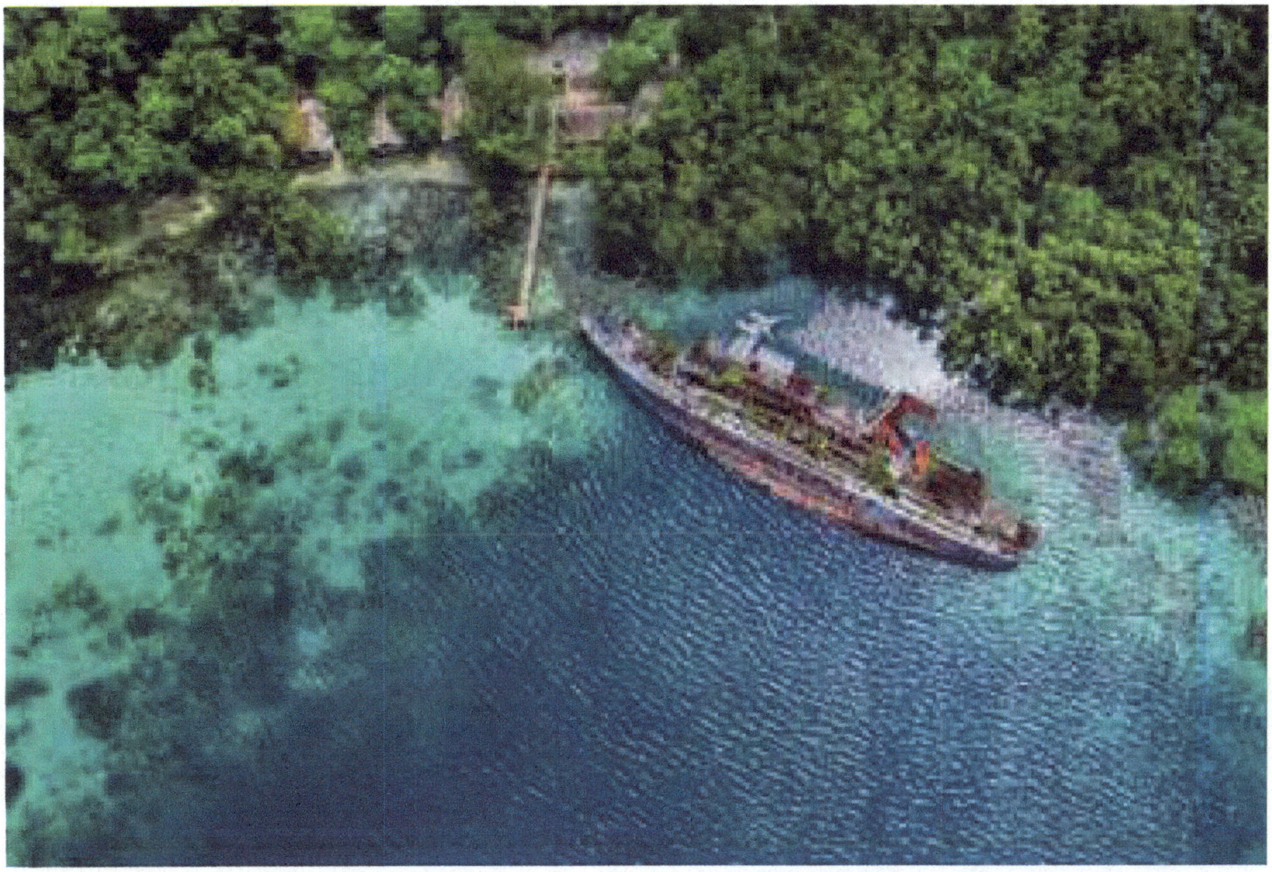

Pumpkin, Coconut and Lime Soup

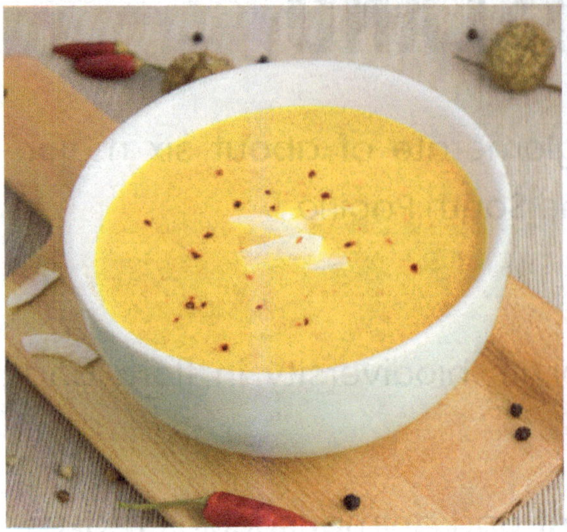

Amount of calories per serving of Pumpkin, coconut and lime soup is 84 calories.

INGREDIENTS

- 2 tablespoons oil.
- 4 chalotes.
- 2 tablespoons ground ginger.
- 2 cloves of garlic.
- 800 grams of pumpkin.
- 4 cups of broth. (1 liter aprox).
- 2 cups of water. (480 ml).
- 3 tablespoons of ground curry.
- 1 cup of coconut milk (240 ml).
- lime juice.
- Salt.
- For Broth:
- Some leek leaves.
- 1 clove of garlic.
- 1 chunk of onion.
- 1 chunk of pepper.
- Salt.
- Parsley.

This perfect soup recipe will satisfy all your lunch cravings.
Solomons Islands boasts of an array of mouth watery dishes to make your stay an experience!

DIRECTIONS

1. We prepare a broth by putting the ingredients in a casserole with water. Put fire on high heat and bring it to a boil. Once it reaches boiling point, turn the fire on low heat, then cook for 30 minutes.
2. Cut the chalotes into little pieces, sauté them in a casserole with oil for 3 minutes until they are golden.
3. Add garlic cut into slices together with ginger, sauté 1 more minute.
4. Peel and cut pumpkin into little pieces, Add it to the casserole. Add the cup of broth and cup of water.
5. Put on a high heat until it reaches boiling point, then turn to a low heat and cook covered for 30 minutes until pumpkin is soft.
6. Don't forget to add salt.
7. Make a purée with the help of a blender.
8. Add curry, coconut milk and lime juice.
9. Stir well and serve with some basil on the top

EUROPE

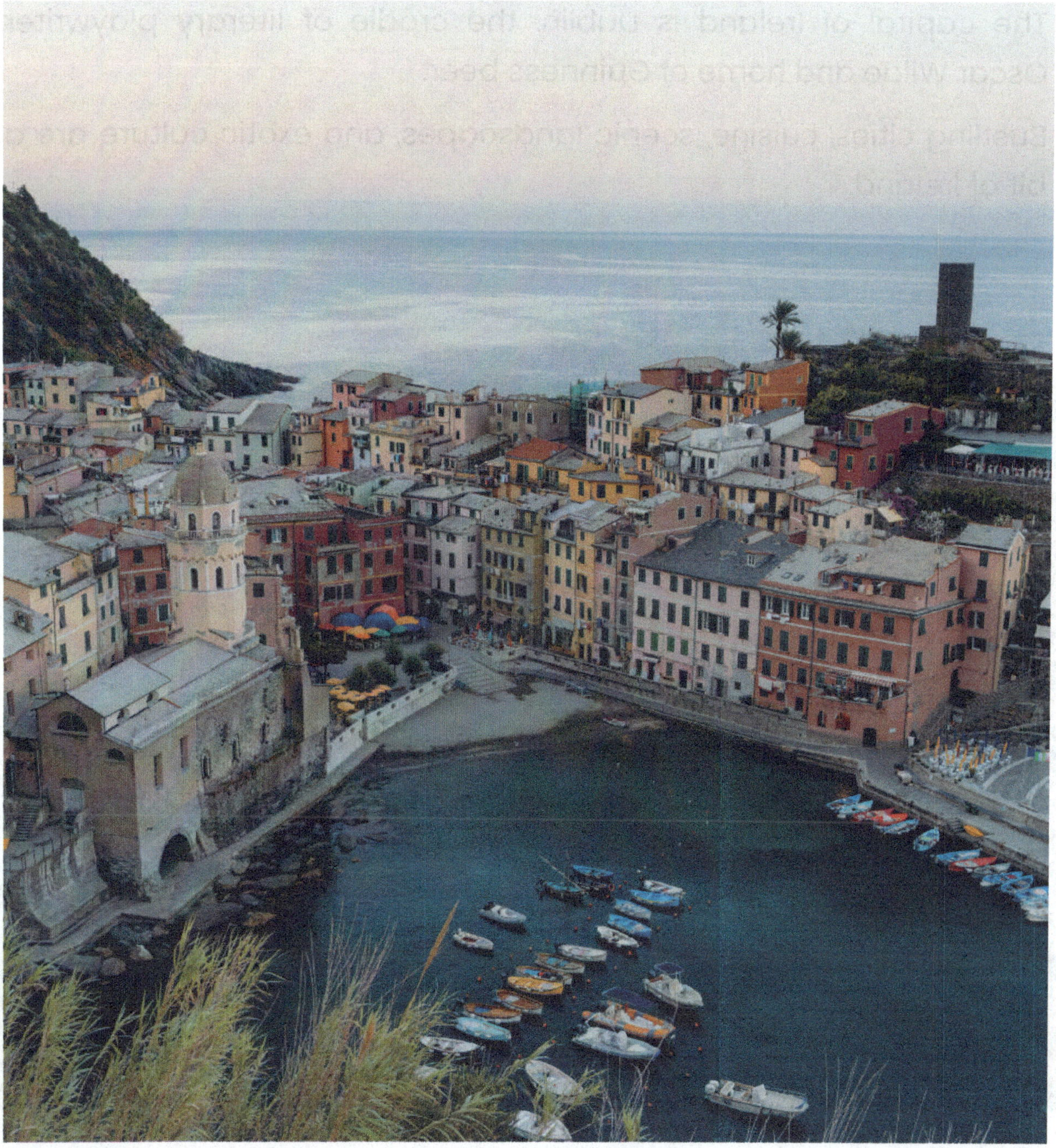

IRELAND

Ireland isEmerald Isle.

This Island in Europe boasts of above 5 million people currently.

The capital of Ireland is Dublin, the cradle of literary playwriter Oscar Wilde and home of Guinness beer.

Bustling cities, cuisine, scenic landscapes, and exotic culture are a bit of Ireland.

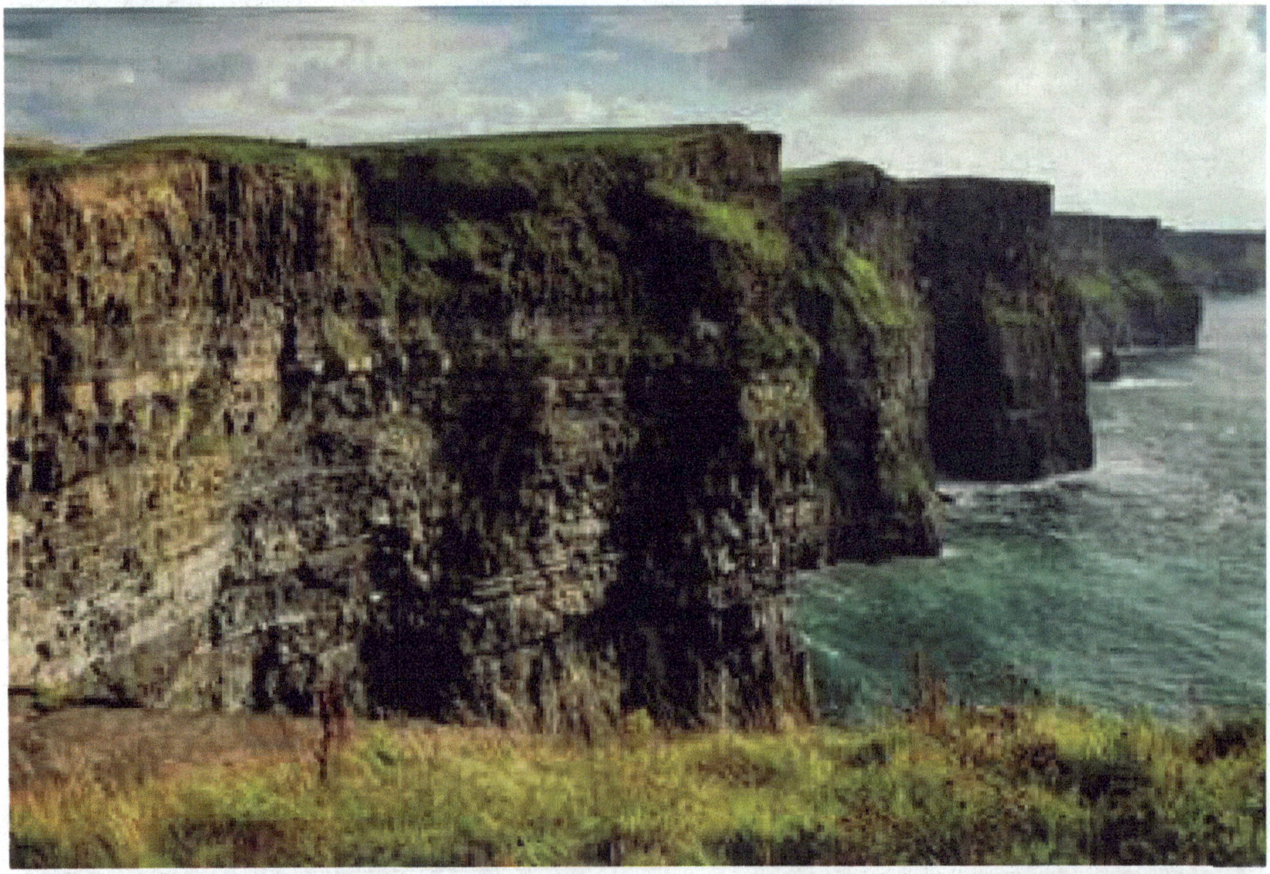

Simple Irish Seafood Chowder Recipe

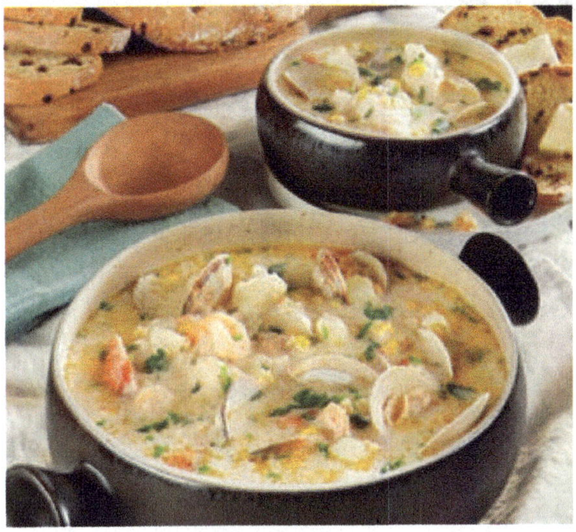

Irish seafood chowder is a traditional soup. In fact, it is Ireland's national soup It a popular Irish dish made with cream and seafood.

INGREDIENTS

- 1.2 litres/2 pints fish stock
- 100g/4oz skinless salmon fillet, cubed
- 100g/4oz skinless haddock fillet, cubed
- 50g/2oz butter 1 onion, chopped
- 2 carrots, chopped
- 1 leek, chopped
- 3 celery sticks, chopped
- 1 tsp chopped fresh dill
- 1 tsp crushed peppercorns
- 50g/2oz plain flour
- Salt and freshly ground black pepper
- A little milk (optional)
- Cream and chopped fresh parsley, to garnish

DIRECTIONS

1. Bring the fish stock to a gentle simmer in a large pan and add the salmon and haddock.
2. Cook for a couple of minutes until tender.
3. Transfer to a plate with a slotted spoon. Set aside.
4. Melt butter in a separate large pan over medium heat.
5. Sweat the onion, carrots, leek, and celery for about 10 minutes or until they are softened
6. Add the dill and peppercorns.
7. Cook for a further 5 minutes.
8. Stir the flour into the vegetable mixture and cook for 5 minutes, stirring constantly.
9. Gradually pour in the fish stock, stirring until smooth after each addition.
10. Boil and simmer for 15 minutes until all of the vegetables are completely tender and the liquid is slightly reduced.
11. Season to taste.

Lovers of castles will definitely love Ashford castle. Experience Ireland in a beautiful way by striding down the streets of rafton Street, Dublin.

MOLDOVA

This Eastern European country capital is Chișinău.

Diverse ethnic groups, scenic mountain sides, arts, and history.

Moldova is home to the tastiest of wines in Europe.

Moldovans make wine at home!

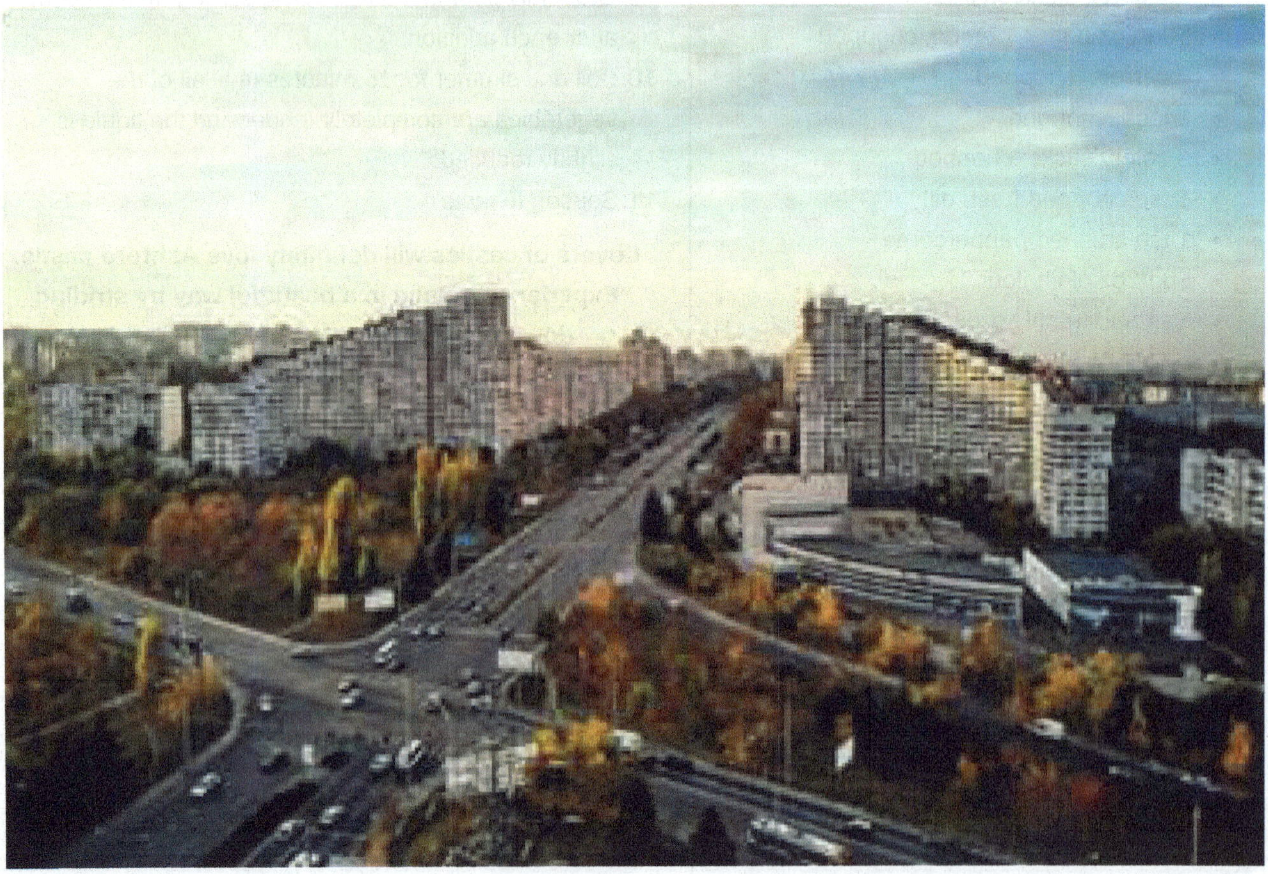

Mondolvan Chicken Soup

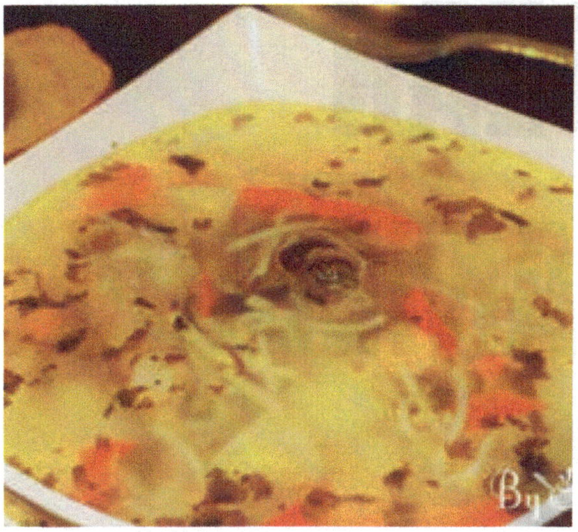

This chicken soup also called Zeamais typical of Moldovans. The hearty protein-rich soup is a must-try on your next visit to Moldova.

INGREDIENTS

- Chicken - about 2 lb (1 kg)
- parsley - 1 root
- onions - 1 head
- carrots - 1
- celery - 1 piece
- potatoes - 12.5 oz (350 g)
- water - 8 1/3 cups (2 L)
- vinegar - 1 tsp
- milk - 1 tbsp
- butter - 1 tbsp
- dill - 1 bunch, can use parsley
- black pepper
- salt

DIRECTIONS

1. Put the cleaned chicken and its offal in a pot with cold water to boil.
2. Shortly after, add the chopped and fried butter onions, celery, carrots, parsley root, and vinegar.
3. Boil on low heat until softened. Strain and let the broth cool, remove the grease.
4. Bring the broth to a boil once again, add the chopped potatoes, and black pepper and keep boiling until they soften.
5. Pour in the milk, and cream, add the meat, and heat it up. Before serving, sprinkle the soup with finely chopped dill or parsley.

An experience of Moldovan wine is an experience of the finest, tastiest and excellently brewed wine in the entire world.

CARIBBEAN & CENTRAL AMERICA

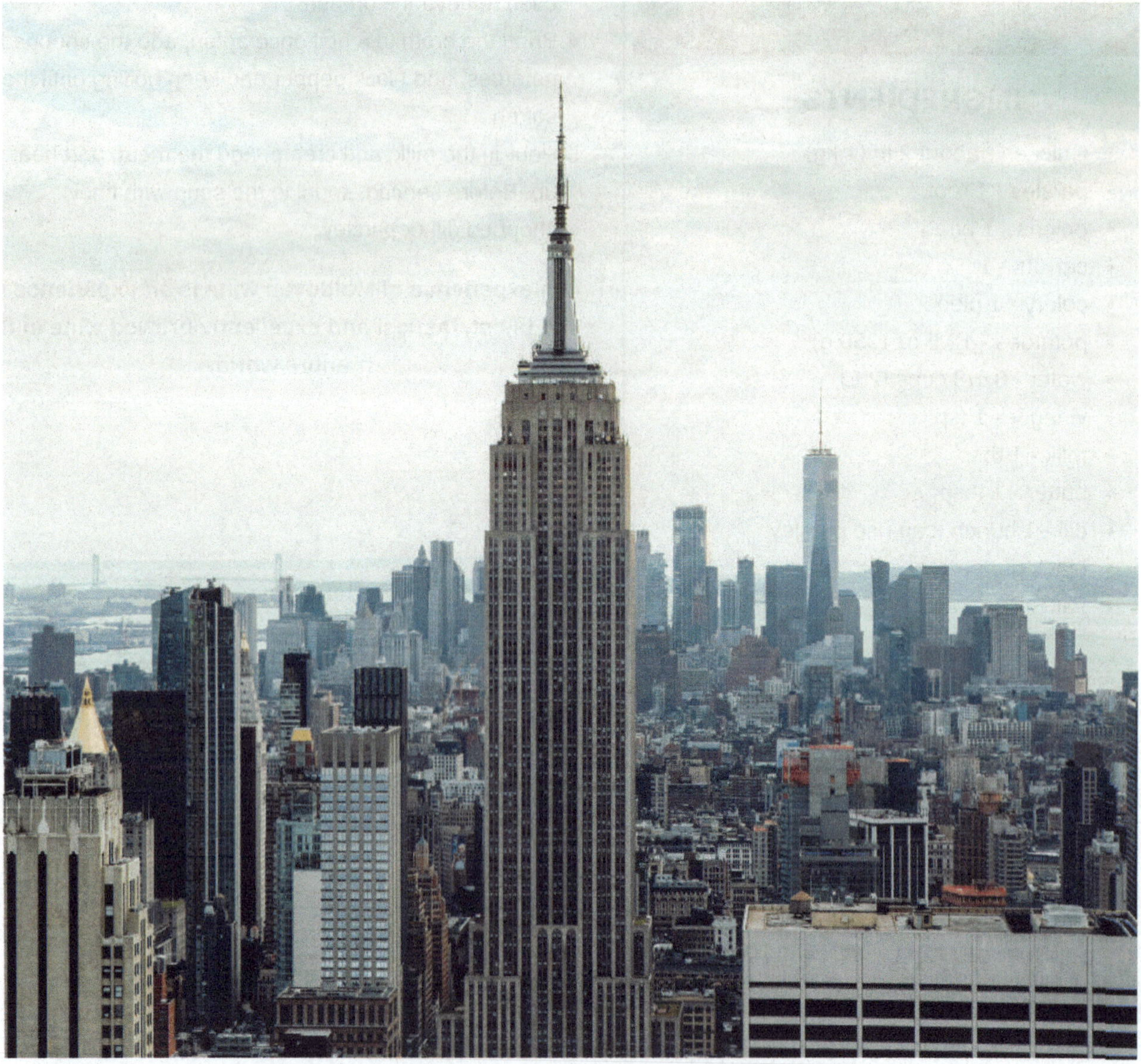

GRENADA

A lover of nutmeg spice? Let's meet here in Grenada!

This Caribbean nation has been nicknamed "Spice Isle".

This mountainous Island with a population of 113,366 persons has its capital in St. George's.

Exotic bars and resorts and pristine beaches are a bit of Grenada.

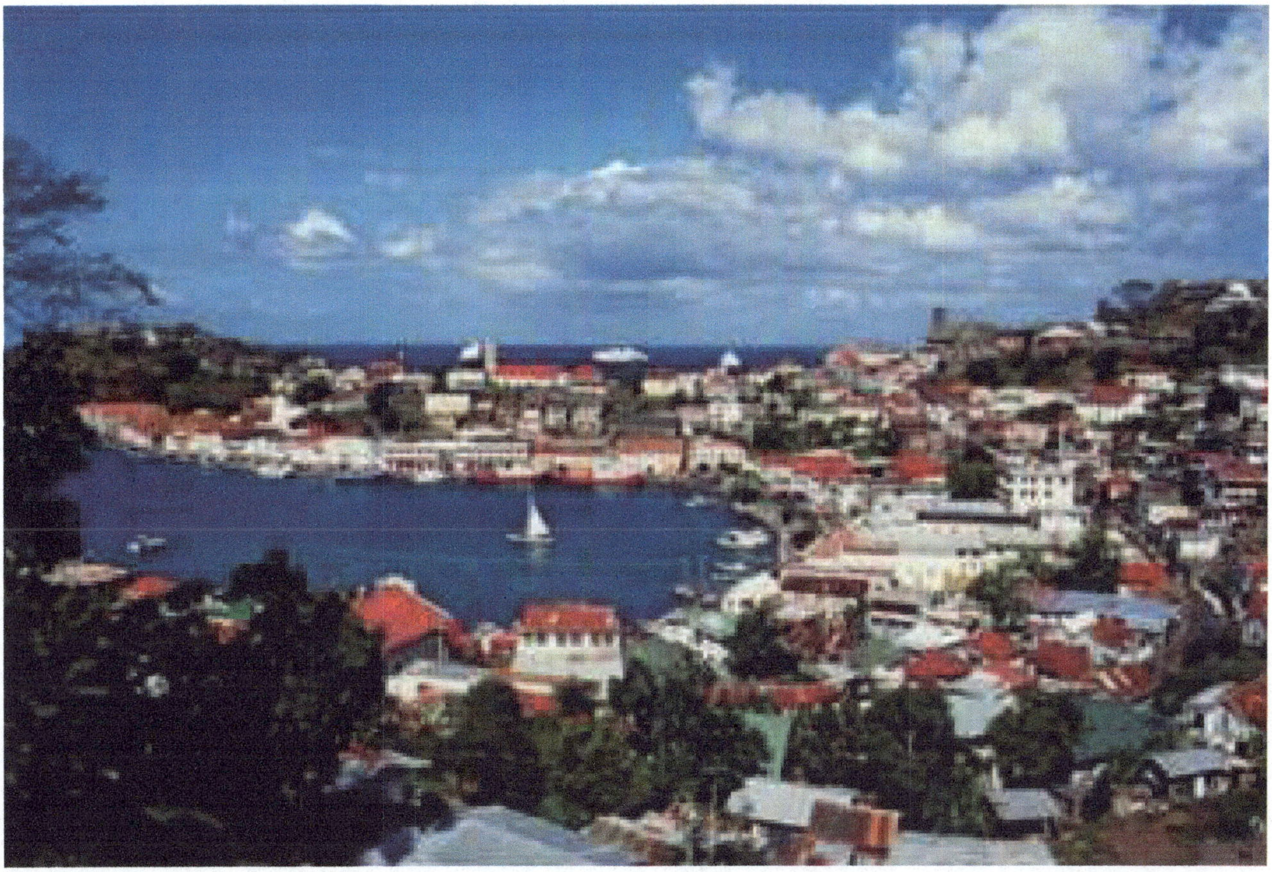

Grenadian Calloo Soup

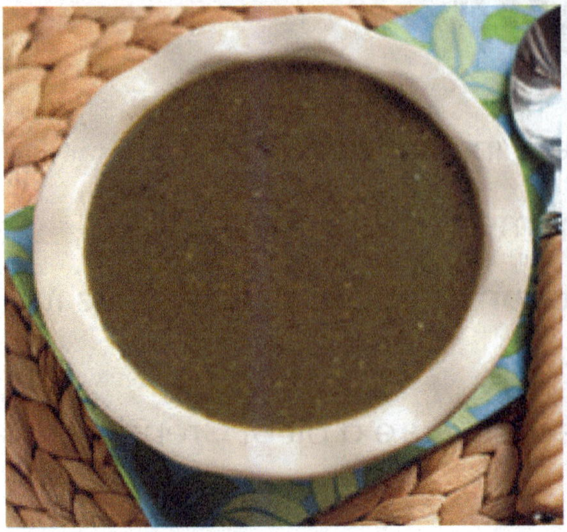

Amount of calories per serving is 544 calories.

INGREDIENTS

- 1 tablespoon canola oil
- 1 medium onion, chopped
- 2 small shallots, roughly chopped
- ¼ cup celery leaves (optional)
- 4-6 cloves roasted garlic, minced
- 1 teaspoon grated fresh ginger
- 2 cans chicken or vegetable stock
- 1 can lite coconut milk
- 1 pound fresh spinach
- 8 ounces cut frozen okra
- ½ teaspoon freshly ground nutmeg
- ½ teaspoon f ground coriander
- ½ teaspoon red chili flakes
- Salt and pepper, to taste

This Caribbean green soup speaks highly of Grenada. Grab your spoon and let's dig in.

DIRECTIONS

1. Heat oil in a large stockpot over medium-high heat and add onion and shallot; cook until slightly soft, about 5 minutes.
2. Add celery (if using), garlic, ginger, stock, and coconut milk and stir together. Add spinach, okra, nutmeg, coriander, and chili flakes and bring to a boil.
3. Reduce heat, and simmer for 30-40 minutes.
4. Puree with a stick blender or in a traditional blender and season with salt and pepper to taste.

A visit to the state capital (Saint George's) to sample the delights of the Underwater Sculpture Park in St. George is a worthy choice!

ST. MAARTEN

This Island in the Caribbean Sea is home to bustling resort beaches and closed coves.

The Island is also known for delicious French cuisine.

A boat cruise across Orient Bay is a must-try.

Lovers of gold, casinos, making, fruit punches, and bustling nightlife.

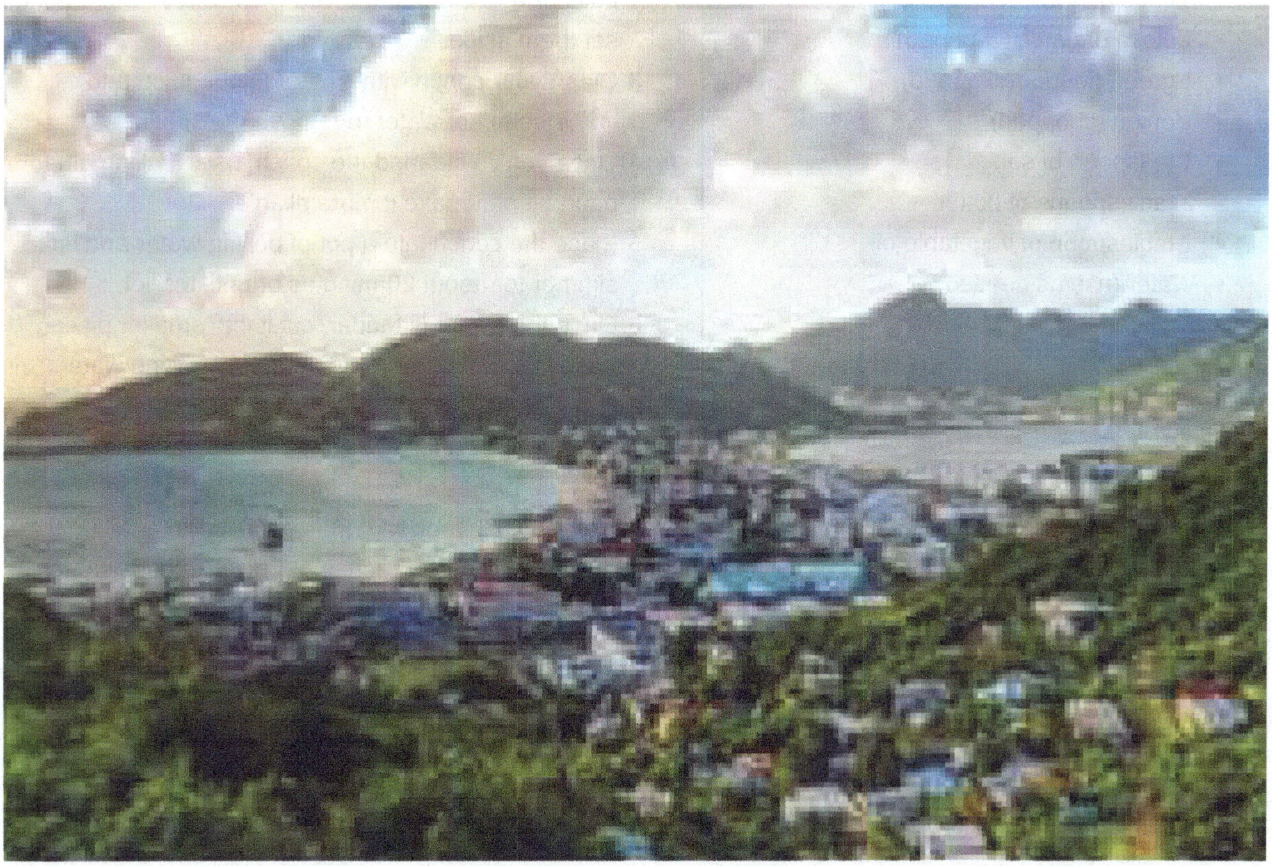

Conch & Dumplings Soup Recipe

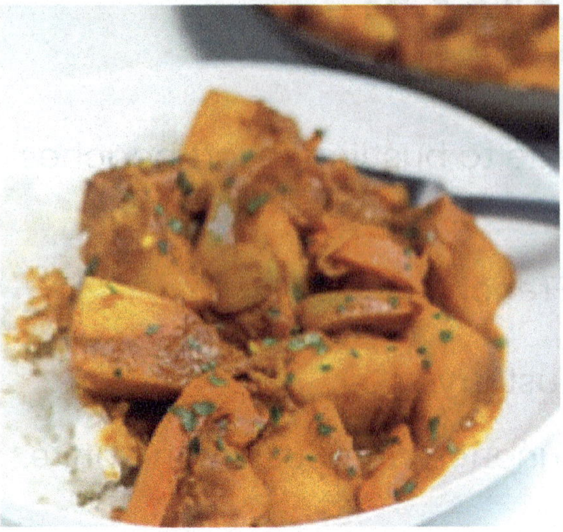

Amount of calories per serving is 737calories.

INGREDIENTS

- 3 pounds of conch
- 4 cups of flour
- 1 clove of garlic (chopped)
- 1 green pepper (chopped)
- 1 onion (chopped)
- 1 teaspoon of salt
- 2 tablespoons of butter
- 1 tablespoon of vegetable oil
- Water (use as needed)

The national dish of Dutch Saint Maarten is the conch and dumplings. First, they pound the conch (sea snail) to tender it—afterward, it's pressure-cooked with dumplings, herbs, and spices. The thick sauce from the conch and dumplings is used as gravy to eat with rice, vegetables, and johnnycakes. You might also find a delicious soup variety of this dish.

DIRECTIONS

1. Mix the flour, sugar, salt, vegetable oil, and butter together. Knead the dough with your hands until you have a smooth and firm mix. Add water as needed. The dough shouldn't stick to your hands, add more flour if it does.
2. Separate pieces of dough and roll them into small balls or whatever shape you wish. Once you're done, set them aside.
3. Clean your conch with lime or lemon juice and immerse in hot water to remove the smell.
4. Once you've cleaned the conch, use a rolling pin to pound it and make it more pliable.
5. Place the conch into a pot of boiling water and let it simmer for about 20 minutes or until tender.
6. Once the conch is tender, cut it into smaller pieces and place them back into the pot of boiling water. Stir in the garlic, pepper, and onion and let it cook for an additional 10 minutes.
7. Add the pieces of dough you set aside earlier to the pot and let it cook with the conch for an additional 10 minutes or until it reaches a gravy-like consistency.
8. Serve hot and enjoy!

A visit to St. Maarten's Maho beach, sipping a chilled glass of guava berry liquors (rum).

SOUTH AMERICA

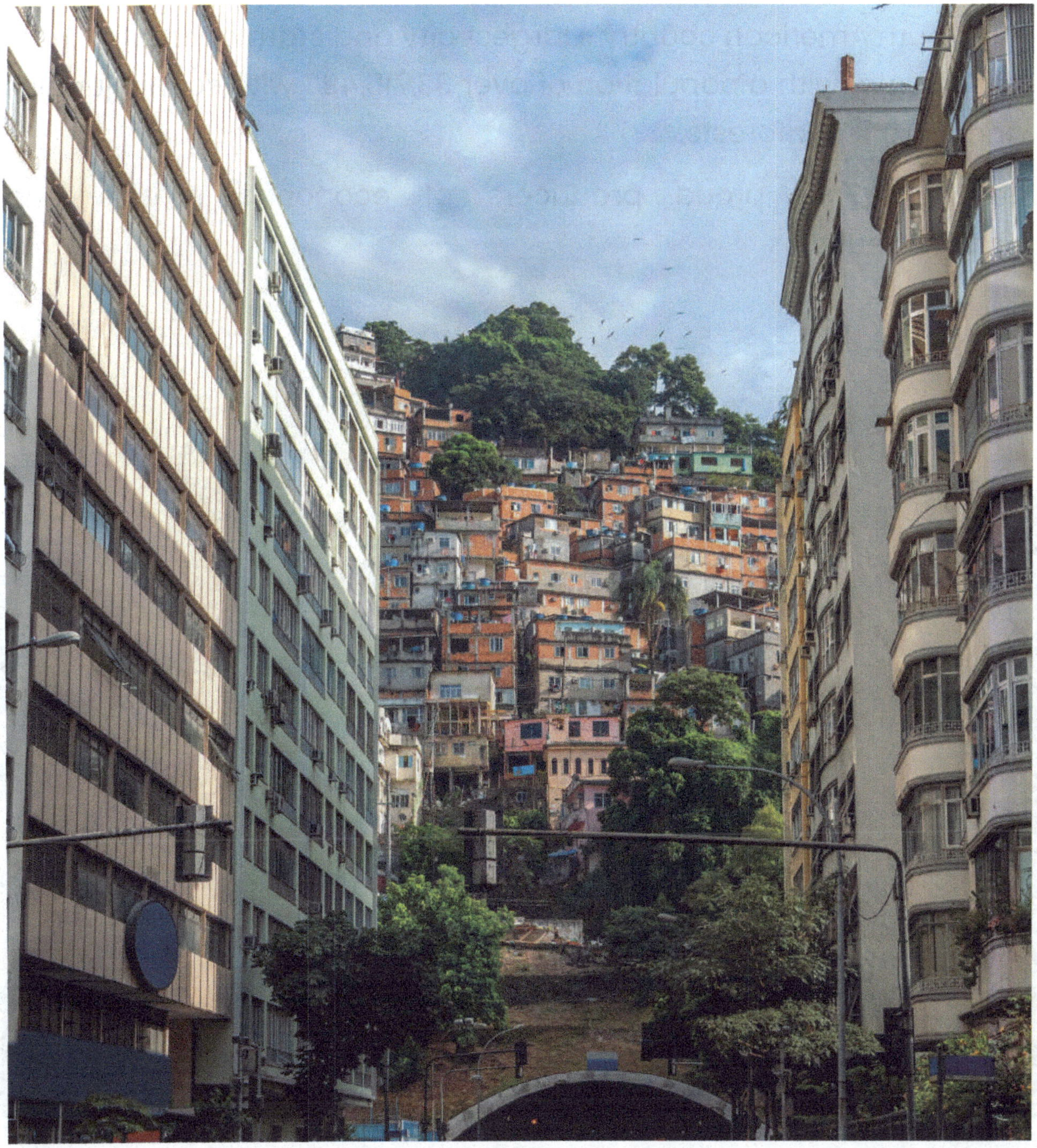

PERU

Also known as the Republic of Peru, dubbed the gastronomic capital of South America.

The South American country's largest city and state capital is Lima. The country with a population of over 33,715,493 with scenic jungles and vibrant rainforests.

Peruvians are proud producers of economic metals and pharmaceuticals.

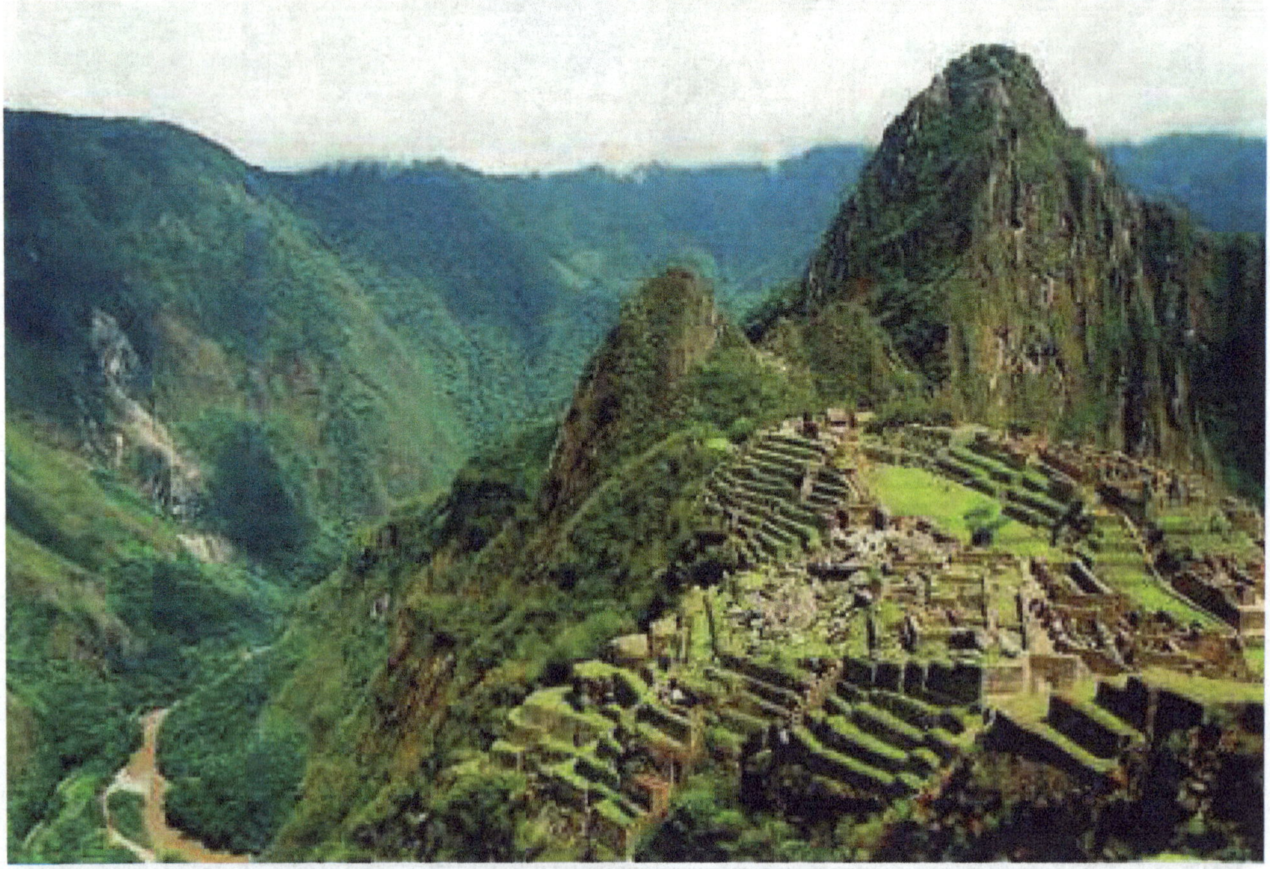

Aji de Gallina (Peruvian Chicken Soup)

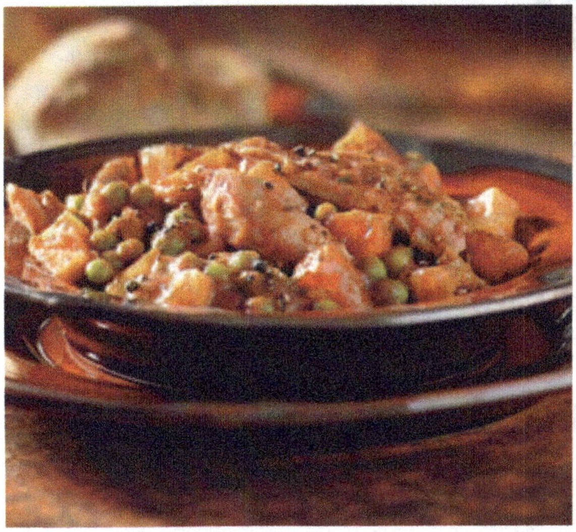

Amount of calories per serving is 488 calories.

INGREDIENTS

- 1 Chicken Breast
- 1 large onion
- 3 garlic cloves
- 3 Peruvian Yellow Peppers
- 1/2 cup Evaporated Milk
- 4 Walnut halves
- 2 slices sandwich Bread
- 2 tablespoons parmesan cheese
- Salt
- Pepper
- black olives
- 1 cooked Egg

You have a thing for birds?
Peru is home to the largest flying bird on earth (the Giant Andean Condor).

Aji de Gallina is a gastronomic fusion of different cultures that gives life to this delicious Peruvian creole dish.
It consists of a soup made of milk, chicken, rice, and many other ingredients that provide a pleasant spicy, and delicious flavor.
The texture and softness of the chicken allow for an explosion of tastes as it enters your mouth.
The wide range of ingredients results in an exquisite broth that has buried itself deep in the hearts of anyone who's tasted it.

DIRECTIONS

1. Cook the entire chicken breast in a pot of water, without salt or anything. Once ready, put the broth aside for later and let the breast cool. When the chicken breast has cooled off, shred it with your hands and save it for later.
2. Make a paste with the yellow pepper by removing the seeds and veins and, with a little bit of the chicken broth, liquefying it until it has a creamy texture; then set it aside.
3. Heat a deep pan and sauté the garlic and onion previously chopped into small pieces. Then add the yellow pepper paste and mix it all, adding some salt and pepper.
4. In another bowl add the bread crumbs with a little of the chicken broth until you have a thick mixture.
5. Add this dough to the pan with the sauce. Stir well and add the ground walnuts and the shredded chicken breast.
6. Add 1 cup of the broth and lower the heat to cook it slowly.
7. After 5 minutes add the Parmesan cheese and let it cook for another 5 minutes.
8. If it has thickened a lot, you can add more broth, if it is too watery, you can add more cheese.
9. After 10 minutes, remove from the heat, add the evaporated milk and stir it well. Then serve with black olives, white rice, and slices of the cooked egg.

BRAZIL

Brazil is the sixth most populous country in the world, having about 215,000000 people.

This largest country in South America. Your stay in Brazil is incomplete without an experience of the Carnival festival.

Samba dance, soccer, and rich cultural heritage are typical of Brazil

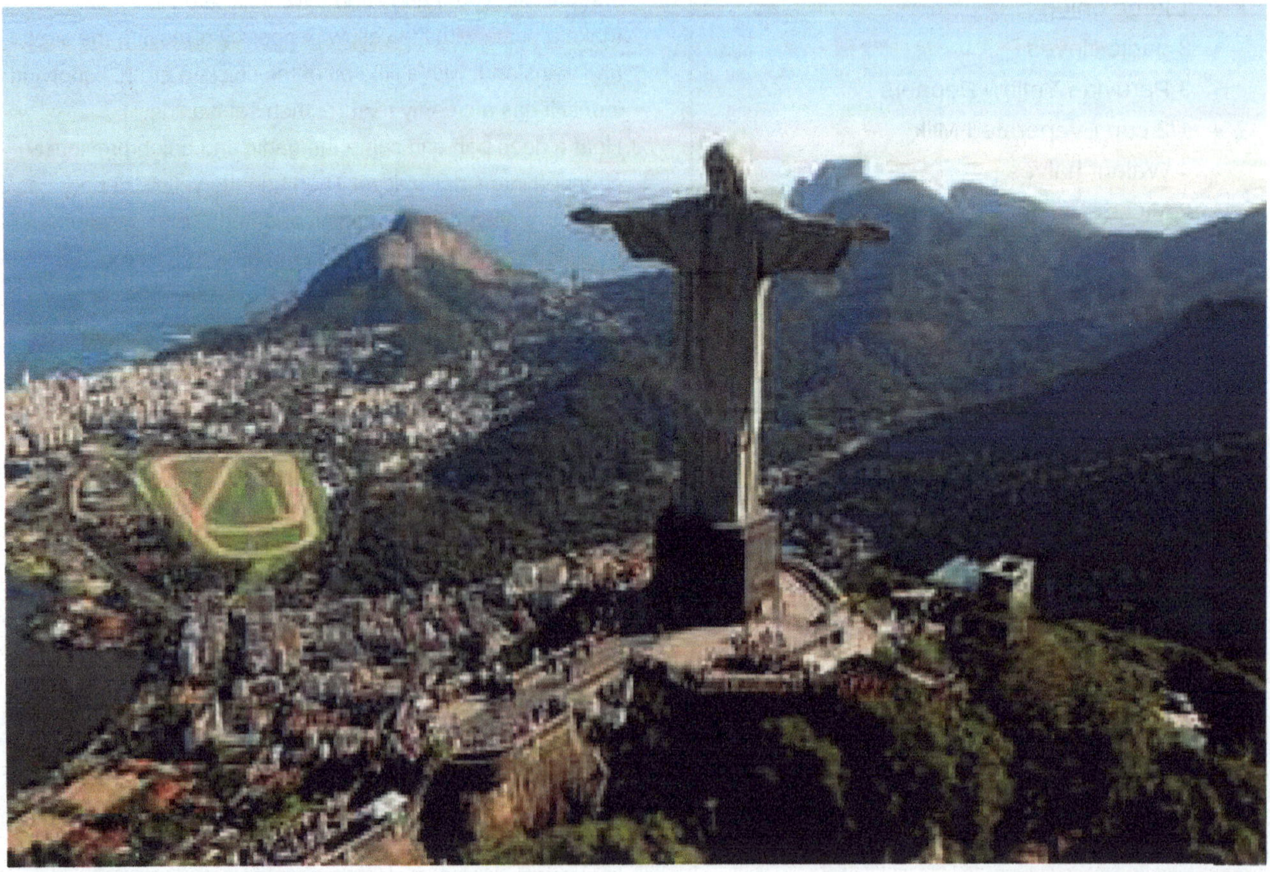

Brazilian Black Bean Soup

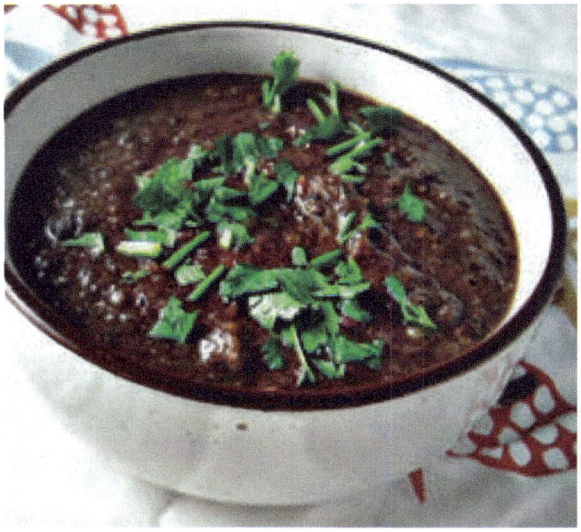

Amount of calories per serving is 522 calories.

INGREDIENTS

- 1 pound (450g) dry black beans
- 4 tablespoons extra virgin olive oil
- 1 pound (450g) pork shoulder
- 2 large onions, sliced
- 1 head garlic, peeled and chopped
- 1 pound (450g) carne seca or corned beef, cut into chunks
- 1/2 pound (225g) fresh sausages, such as chorizo or Italian sausage
- 1 pound (450g) smoked sausage, such as linguica or kielbasa
- 1 smoked ham hock or shank
- 3 to 4 bay leaves
- Water
- 1 14.5 ounce can (411g) crushed tomatoes
- Kosher salt

A chilled glass of cachaça (an alcohol distillate from sugarcane) on the sandy beaches of Brazil is an experience you will never forget!

Brazil's cuisine often features smoky, grilled meats, but this healthy vegetarian bean soup recipe is completely meat-free.
Instead, blackened jalapeños, fire-roasted tomatoes, and smoked paprika provide the Brazilian flair.
Black beans are a perfect lunch recipe if you want it to be authentically Brazilian. A Portuguese version uses white beans.

DIRECTIONS

1. Soak the beans in hot water:
2. Pour boiling water over the black beans and let them sit while you prepare the rest of the stew.
3. Brown the pork shoulder:
4. Heat the olive oil in a large pot over medium-high heat and brown the pork shoulder. When the meat has browned, remove the meat from the pot, set aside.
5. Brown the onions and add garlic:
6. Add the onions to the pot. Brown them, stirring occasionally, scraping up any browned bits from the bottom of the pot.
7. Sprinkle a little salt over the onions and add the garlic. Stir well and sauté 2 more minutes.
8. Add the meat, bay leaves, and water:
9. Add back the pork shoulder and the other meats. Add enough water to cover all ingredients. Add the bay leaves, cover, and bring to a simmer. Cook gently for 1 hour.
10. Add the soaked black beans:
11. Drain the black beans from their soaking liquid and add them to the stew. Simmer gently, covered, until the beans are tender, about an hour and a half.
12. Add the tomatoes, stir well and taste for salt, adding if it's needed. Simmer this, uncovered, until the meat begins to fall off the ham hock, which will probably take 2 to 3 hours.
13. Serve with white rice and hot sauce. A classic side dish would be sautéed collard greens.

SECTION 1V

DINNER

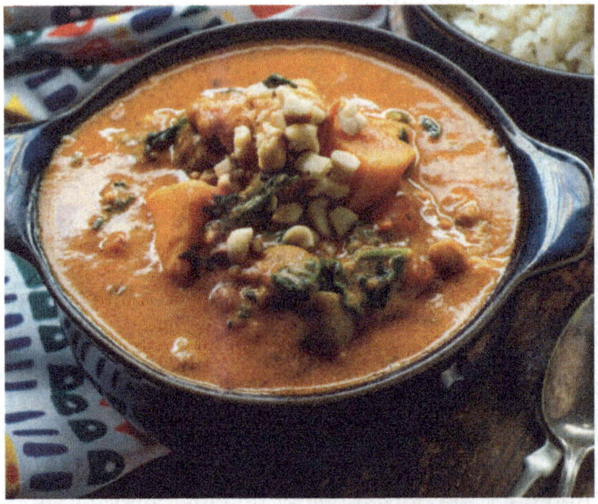

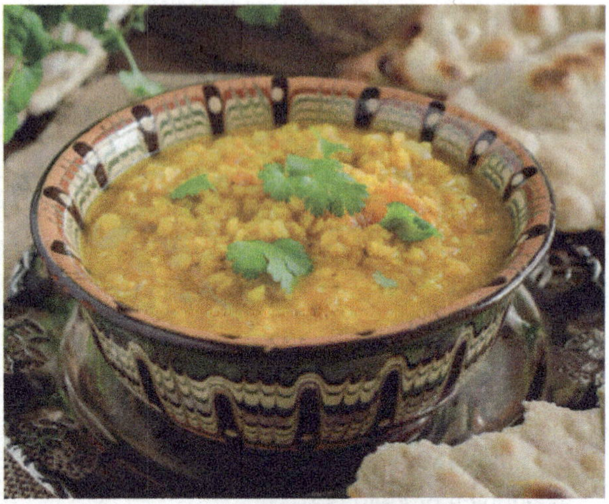

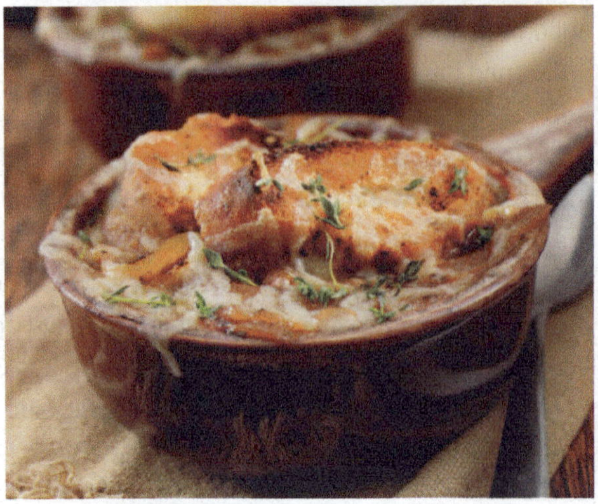

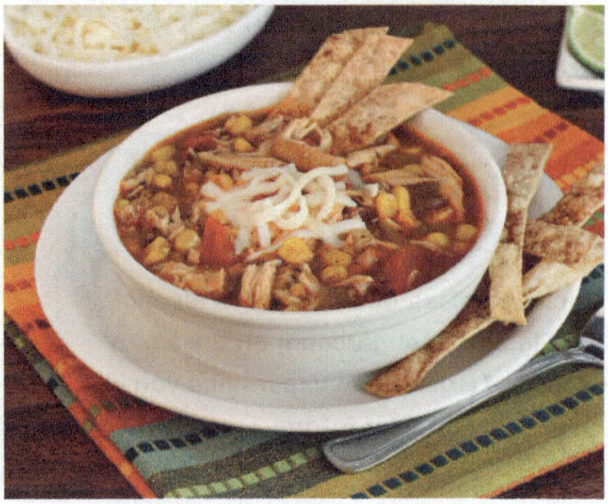

AFRICA

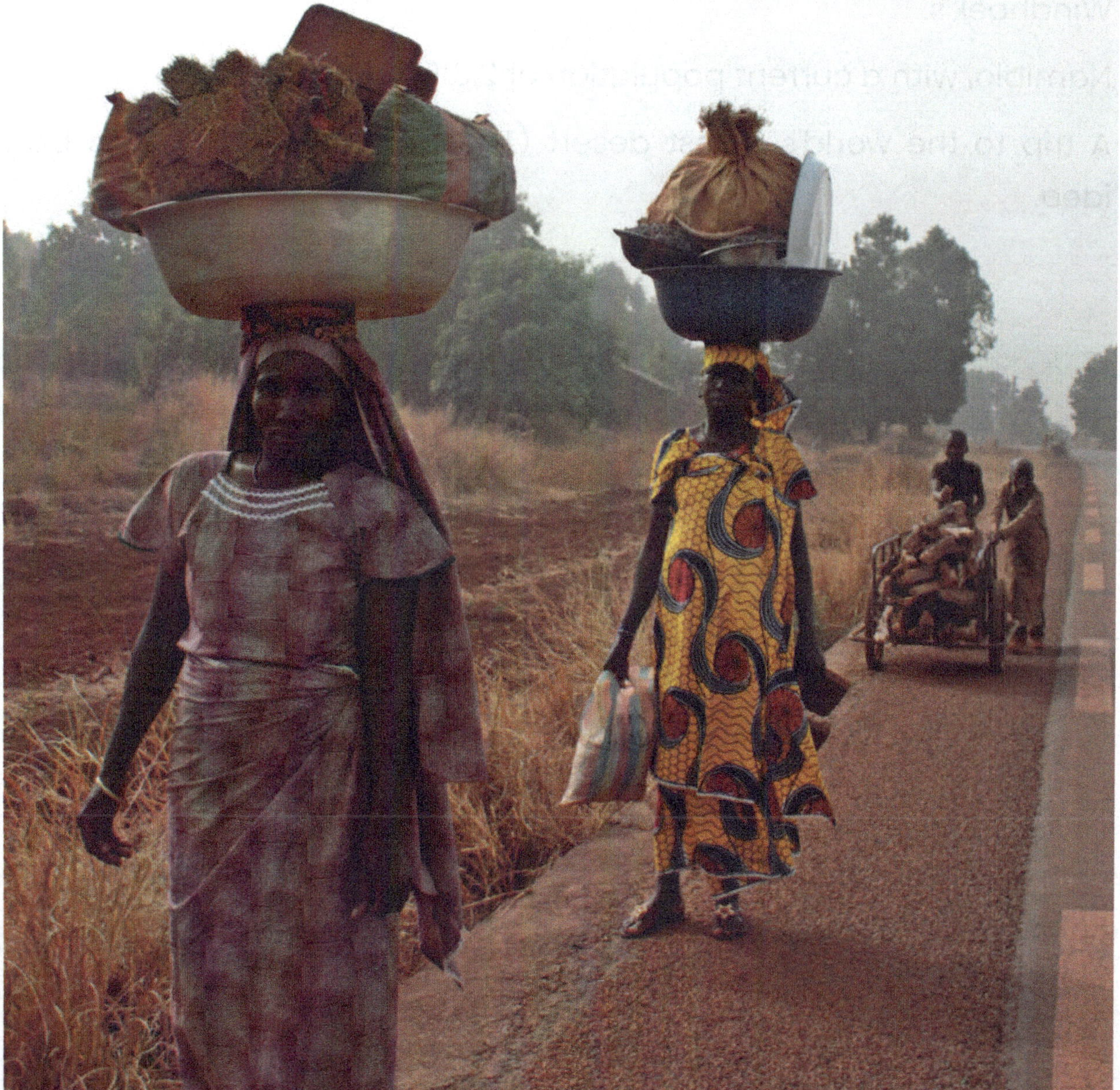

NAMIBIA

This southwest African country boasts a variety of diverse wildlife.

Lovers of cheetah will love it here. Windhoek, the capital city is home to ancient pre-historic German buildings such as Windhoek's.

Namibia, with a current population of 2,615,763.

A trip to the world's oldest desert (The Namib) will not be a bad idea.

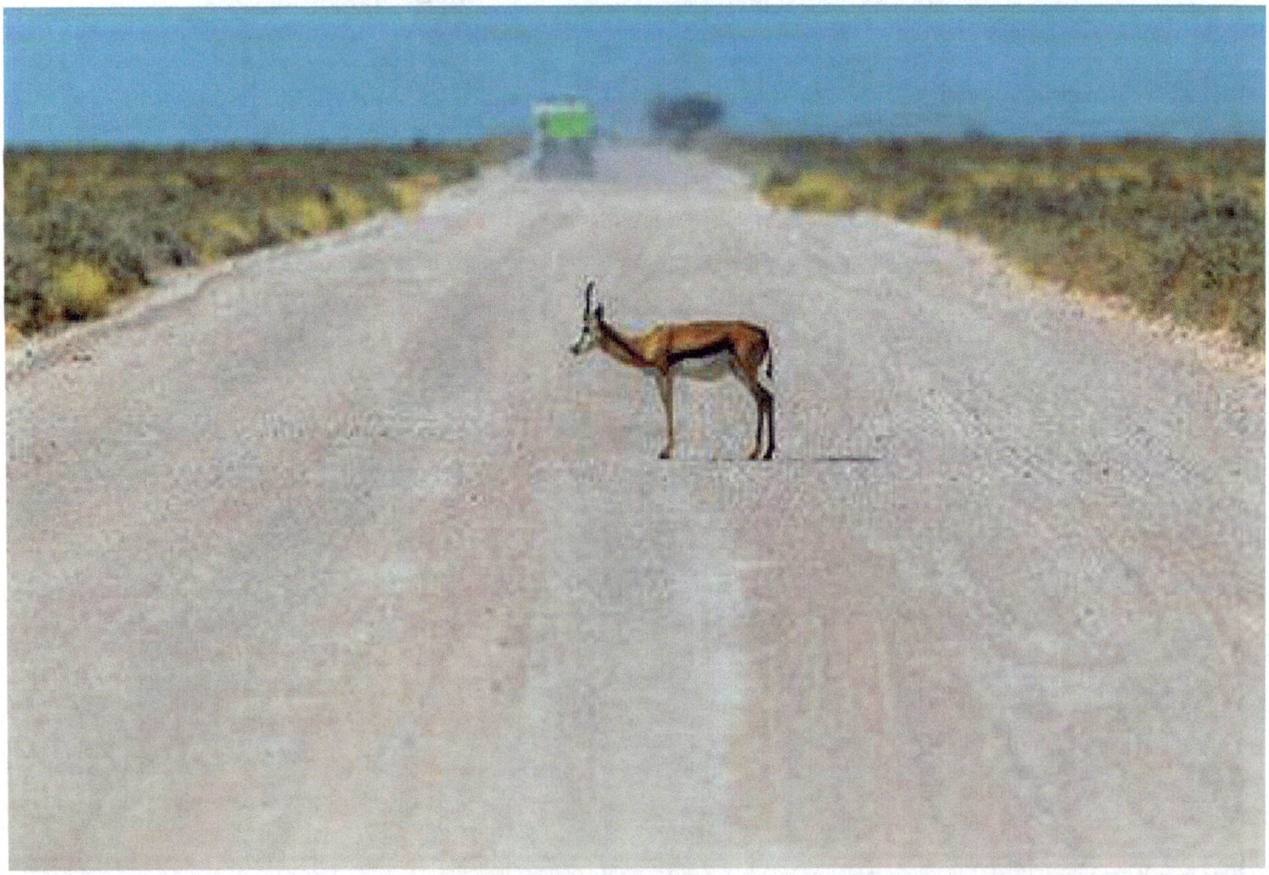

Namibian Peanut Soup

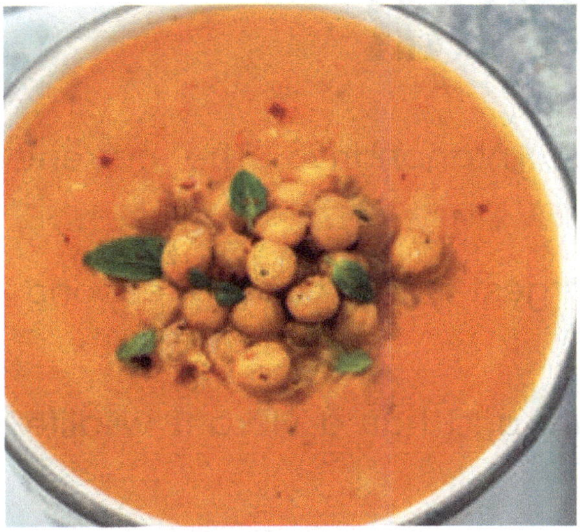

INGREDIENTS

- 1 Cup Peanut
- 1 Tbsp Crayfish
- 1 Smoked Turkey Thigh
- 1 Lb Beef
- 1/4 to 1/2 Cup Peanut Oil
- Handful Spinach
- 1 large Tomato
- 1 Bell pepper
- 1 Large Onion
- 1 Tablespoon Crayfish
- 1 Habanero Pepper
- 2 Seasoning Cubes
- 2 Teaspoons Grated Ginger
- Palm Oil or Peanut Oil

Spicy Peanut soup or Groundnut stew is a staple in most African cuisine in Namibia. It is warm, nourishing, and full of flavors. It is also very versatile which makes it perfect for dinner or lunch.

DIRECTIONS

1. The first thing to do is to wash, season, and boil the beef.
2. Roast the Peanuts for about 5 minutes or until it well browned
3. Use a coffee grinder or a dry mill grinder to grind the peanuts to a fine
4. De-bone the roast Turkey and cut it into bite sizes and add to the boiling beef after about 10 minutes of cooking the meat. Then continue the cooking process for about 30 more minutes or till the meat becomes tender
5. Blend together the peppers, Tomatoes and the other half of the Onion.
6. Add the blended pepper, crayfish, Palm Oil and the ground peanut to the boiling meat and leave to cook for
7. Add the ground peanuts to the stew and mix thoroughly until the peanut is totally dissolved in the stew. Cover it up and leave to cook for about 10 to 12 minutes
8. Stir in the Spinach and leave to simmer for an additional two minutes
9. Serve while still hot over a plate a Rice, Couscous Fonio or swallows like Fufu and pounded yam. Enjoy!

Etosha National Park's salt pan holds a large proportion of Namibia's wildlife excitement, sampling many wildlife giraffes

MADAGASCAR

This East African country'scapital is Antananarivo. The current population is 28,846,522.

Madagascar is the world's second-largest island country, second only to Indonesia.

This nation is home to diverse lemurs and has a vibrant wildlife community.

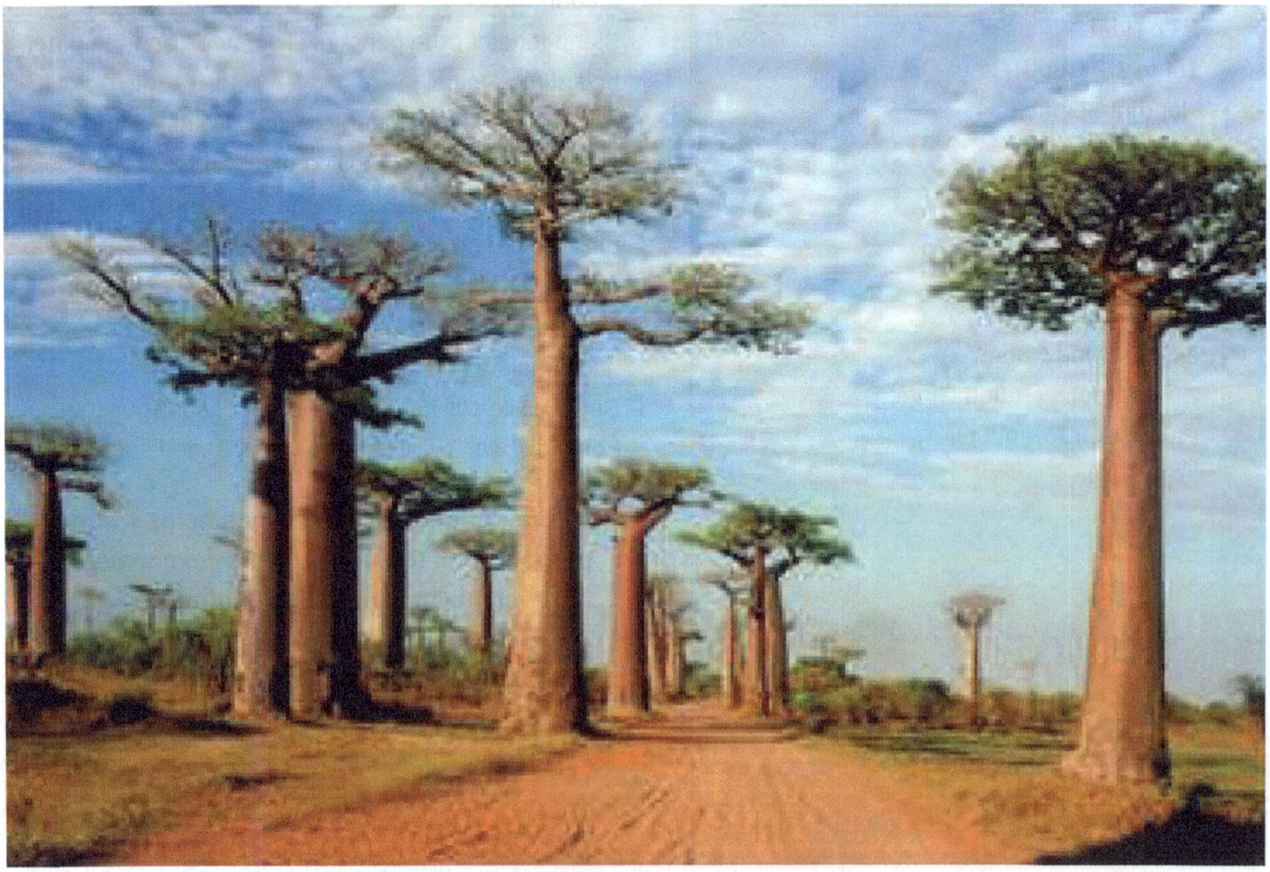

Madagascar's Cabbage Soup

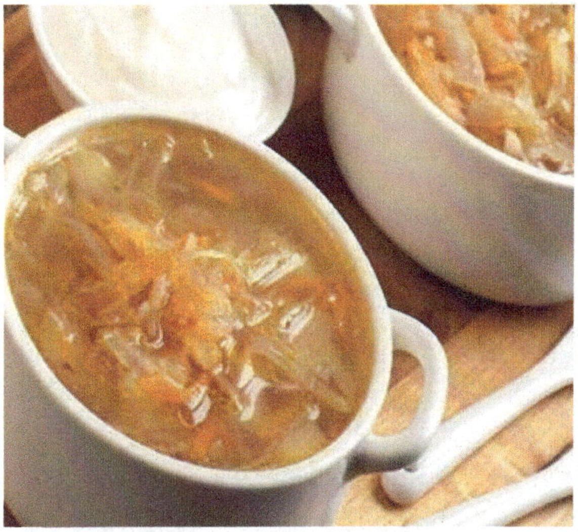

Amount of calories per serving is 155.

INGREDIENTS

- 1 sliced onion
- 3 cloves finely chopped garlic
- 2 tsp ground coriander seeds
- 5 cup veg stock
- 4 diced tomato
- 1 pinch ground salt
- 2 tablespoon butter
- 2 teaspoon jalapeno
- 1 tablespoon mustard seeds
- 2 tablespoons lemon juice
- 1 cup sliced cabbage
- 1 pinch ground black pepper

This is the national dish of Madagascar. This soup dish will surely warm you up on a cold day being prepared with vegetable stock, tomato, cabbage, jalapeno, and onions.

DIRECTIONS

1. Heat ghee or butter in a saucepan over moderate flame. Add sliced onions in the saucepan and sauté them over medium flame till they are golden in color. Once done, add the garlic and jalapeno. Continue to sauté for another two minutes. Add coriander and dry mustard. Stir well.
2. Now add the vegetable stock and tomatoes. Make sure that that the saucepan is uncovered and simmer the ingredients for about 10 minutes. Then add cabbage and cook for another five minutes. Season with salt, pepper and lemon juice. Serve the warm soup with garlic bread.

A sip of ranonapango (overcooked rice water concentrate) is a popular rum amongst the locals.

ASIA

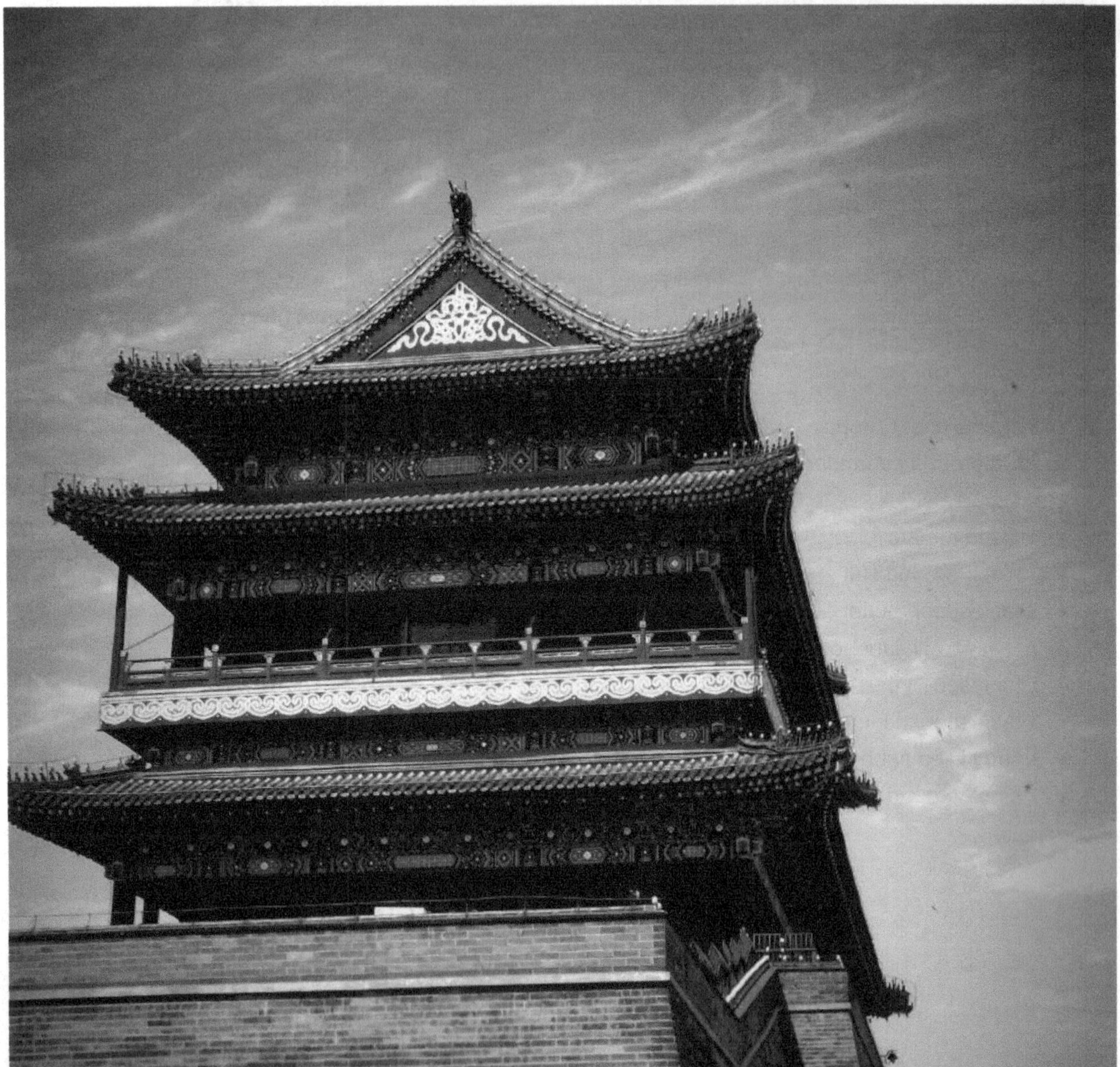

YEMEN

The middle Eastern country was formerly called South Arabia.

This west Asian country's capital and largest city is Sana'a. Clement weather, mud-like houses, and delicious staples are common in Yemen.

With a current population of 30,892,506,
Yemen is host to an abundance of Frankincense and myrrh.

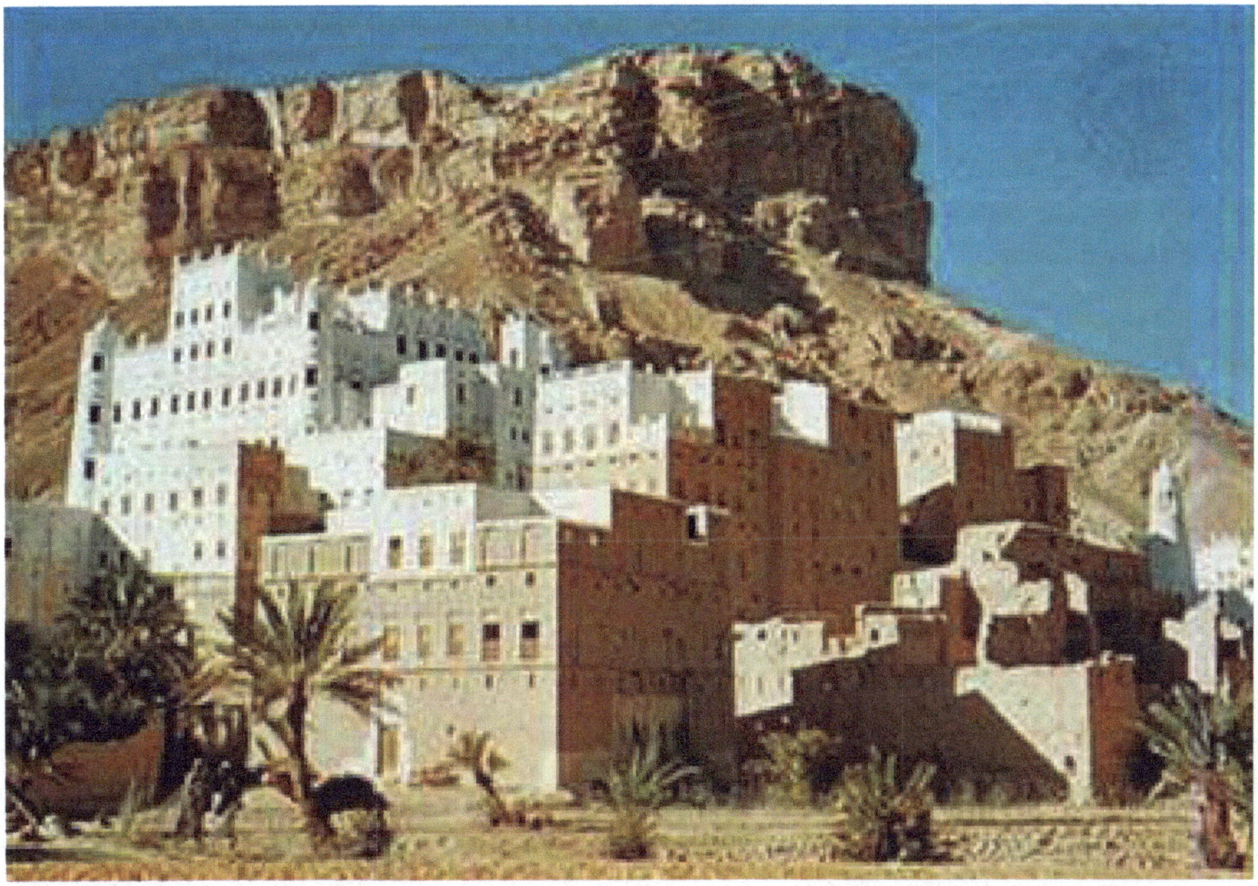

Fahsa Soup Recipe

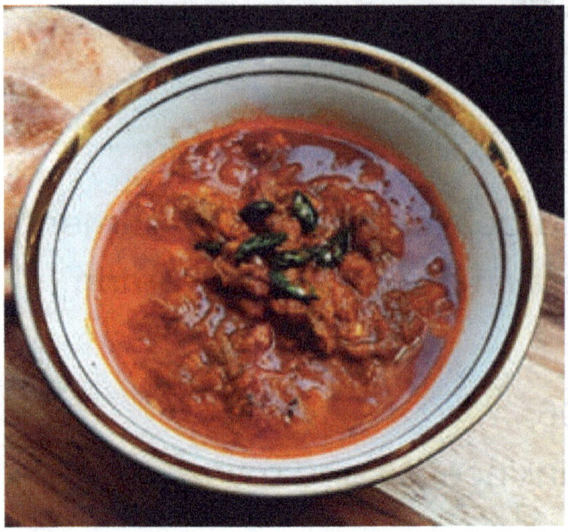

This sweet soup has 3 components, meat broth, spices and herbs, and fenugreek dip). Fahsa is from Yemen, and it's a stew, not just any type of stew, though—it is made with lamb meat.The preparation of the meat broth and fenugreek can happen in succession. But, it will be easier and better if you have already prepared hilbah dip and lamb broth.

INGREDIENTS

- 1 tbsp cooking oil, like canola oil
- 3 cloves of garlic, minced
- 1 lb of lamb cubes
- 5 cups of lamb broth or water
- ½ tsp coriander
- ¼ tsp turmeric
- ½ tsp cumin
- 1 green chili pepper, chopped
- Half a medium-sized onion, finely chopped
- 3 tbsp of hilba, or to taste
- Salt, to taste

DIRECTIONS

1. Add the oil to a pressure cooker over medium heat, then sauté the onions, garlic, and chili pepper.
2. Once the garlic browns and the onions go translucent, add the turmeric, coriander, cumin, salt, and lamb cubes, which should be washed thoroughly.
3. Let the meat cook for about 5 minutes before adding the broth or water, then seal the pressure cooker and leave it for 30 minutes more. Heat should still be on medium.
4. Remove from heat when the meat is fully tender (30 minutes or more duration). Release pressure and allow the cooker to cool before opening.
5. Use a wooden ladle to break up the meat into smaller pieces. This should be easy if your meat is truly tender.
6. Pour the stew into a stoneware pot and heat it up until it bubbles.
7. Add the already-prepared hilba. Then serve hot with bread.

MONGOLIA

The East Asian nation Capital is Ulaanbaatar with a population of 3,363,897.

Mongolia dubbed as "the land of the blue sky" Perhaps a taste of the local Mongolian drink made from fermented mare's milk, airag is known for its therapeutic benefits.

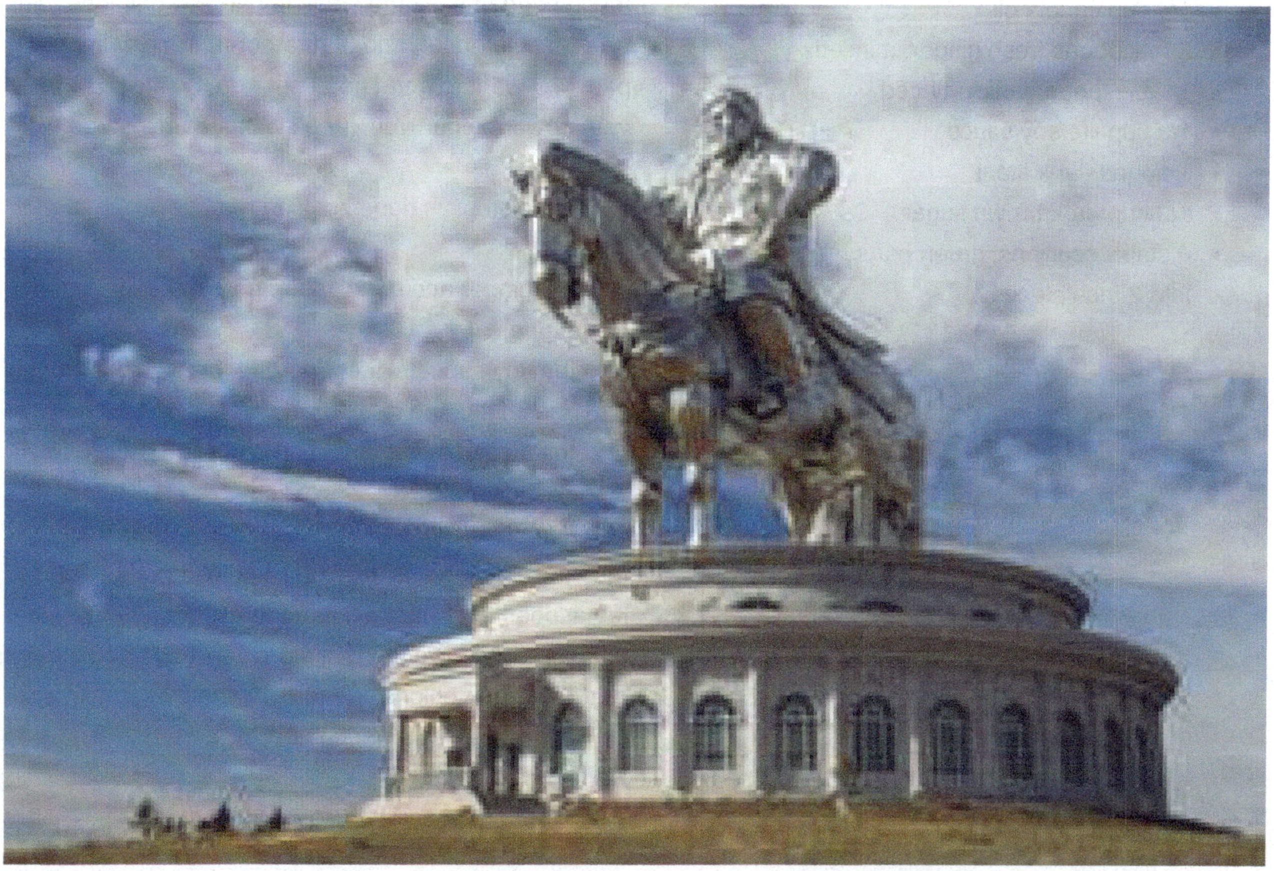

Mongolian Beef Soup

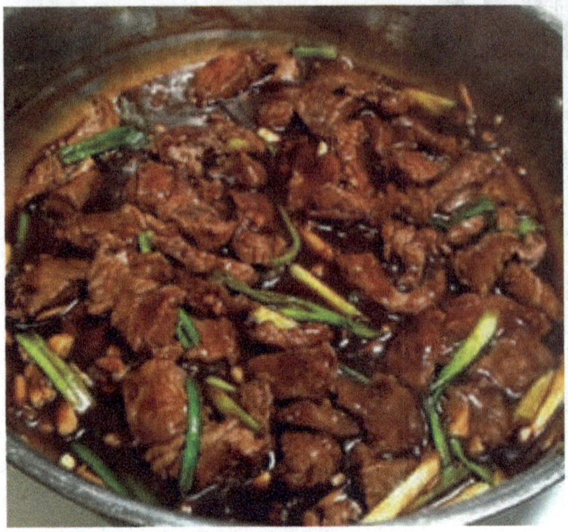

Amount of calories per serving is 433kcal.

Mongolian Beef that's easy to make in just 30 minutes, crispy, sweet and full of garlic and ginger flavors you love from your favorite Chinese restaurant.

INGREDIENTS

- 1/4 cup cornstarch
- 1/4 cup canola oil
- 2 teaspoons fresh ginger, minced
- 1 tablespoon garlic, minced
- 1/3 cup lite soy sauce
- 1 pound flank steak
- 1/2 cup dark brown sugar
- 4 stalks scallions, green parts only, cut into 2-inch pieces

DIRECTIONS

1. Slice the flank steak against the grain (the grain is the length of the steak) the long way ¼ inch think pieces and add it to a ziploc bag with the cornstarch.
2. Press the steak around in the bag making sure each piece is fully coated with cornstarch and leave it to sit.
3. Add the canola oil to a large frying pan and heat on medium high heat.
4. Add the steak, shaking off any excess corn starch, to the pan in a single layer and cook on each side for 1 minute.
5. If you need to cook the steak in batches because your pan isn't big enough do that rather than crowding the pan, you want to get a good sear on the steak and if you crowd the pan your steak with steam instead of sear.
6. When the steak is done cooking remove it from the pan.
7. Add the ginger and garlic to the pan and sauté for 10-15 seconds
8. Add the soy sauce, water and dark brown sugar to the pan and let it come to a boil.
9. Add the steak back in and let the sauce thicken for 20-30 Seconds
10. The cornstarch we used on the steak should thicken the sauce, if you find it isn't thickening enough add 1 tablespoon of cornstarch to 1 tablespoon of cold water and stir to dissolve the cornstarch and add it to the pan.
11. Add the green onions, stir to combine everything, and cook for a final 20-30 Seconds
12. Serve immediately.

OCEANIA

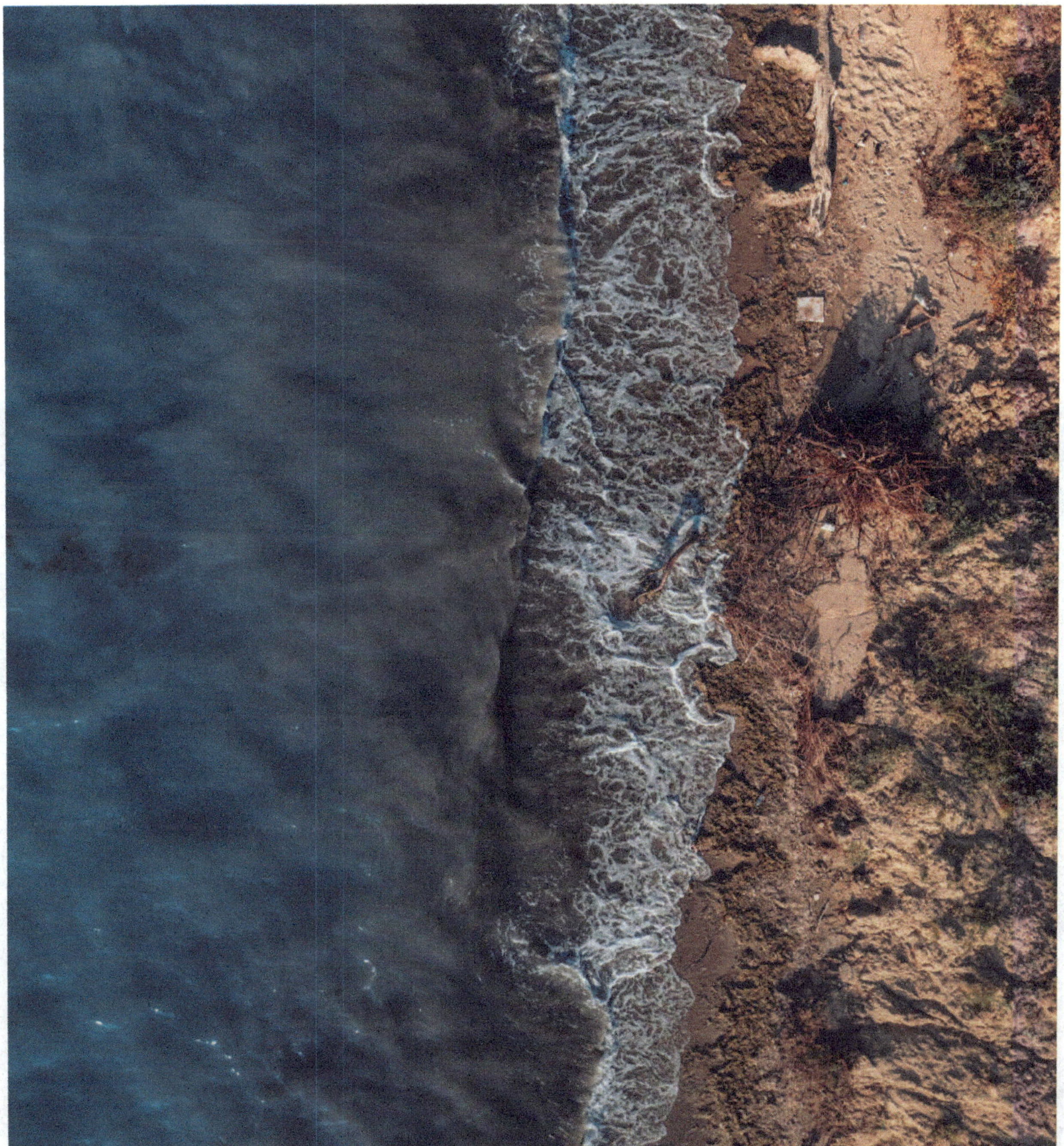

FIJI

With an abundance of islands, palm-fringed beaches, thriving coral reefs, and, Fiji has become a plug for adventure and relaxation.

Traditional Fijian food consists of fresh fish, coconut, root crops, and steamed greens.

A choice dish, roro, is made from steamed taro leaves, onion, garlic, oil, and coconut milk. The result is a comfort food that goes well with just about any Fijian dish. It tastes like a tropical version of creamed spinach.

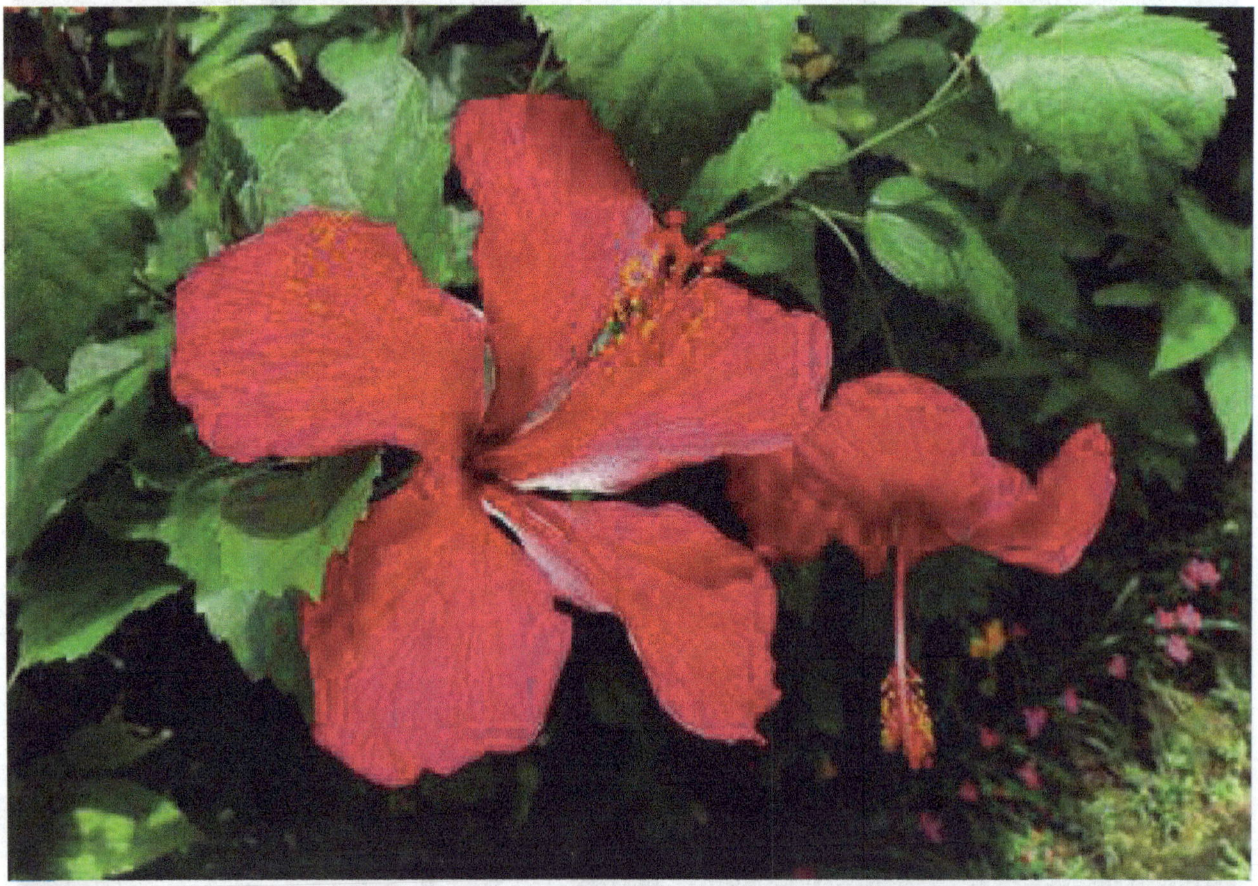

Fijian Dhal Soup

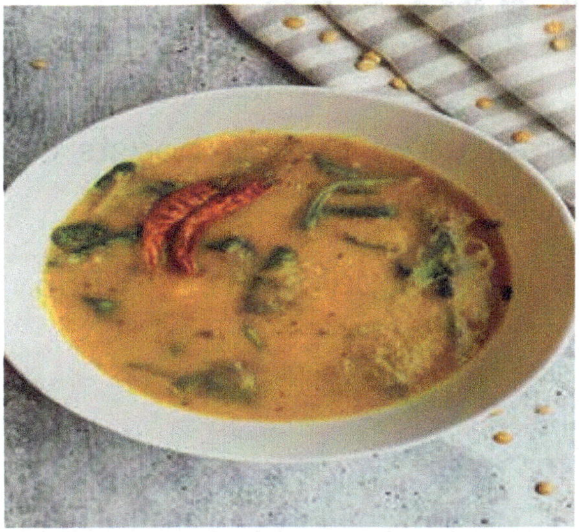

This flavored dhal curry is a lovely dinner soup. An exotic blend of fenugreek seeds, yellow mustard seeds, garlic, crushed chili pepper, turmeric in a one pot soup.

INGREDIENTS

- 1 tbsp ghee
- 1/4 tsp turmeric
- 1-2 green Thai chili peppers
- 1/2 tbsp garlic cloves minced
- 1/2 yellow onion sliced
- 1/2 cup yellow split peas or any lentil toor, masoor, mung, moong, uraddals
- 1 whole carrot peeled and sliced into rounds
- 1 tomato diced
- 2 cups Water
- 1 tsp kosher salt
- 4 ounces spinach

DIRECTIONS

1. Add in all ingredients for the Instant Pot Dhal except the spinach. Stir all ingredients. Close pot with lid.
2. Select Pressure Cook (Hi) and adjust the pressure cook time to 5 minutes. Allow 5 minutes of natural pressure release and then release the remaining pressure manually.
3. While the dhal is cooking, heat ghee in a fry pan. Add 3-seed mixture, onions, garlic and curry leaves until golden. Turn off heat
4. Open instant pot once pressure is release, if more water is needed, you can add 1/2 a cup now. Cook on sauté mode. Mix in fried tadka mix.
5. Use immersion blend to pulse ingredients together. Once you are a consistency you like, mix in spinach. Once dhal starts to bubble you can turn off the instant pot.

Catch the Fijian fever at theMamanuca Islands, for a taste of the rich Fijian culture and step down your favorite dessert with the Kava drink to calm your nerves.

FRENCH POLYNESIA

French Polynesia, an overseas conglomerate of France, boasts of over 90 Islands, sandy beaches, epic waterfalls.

The capital city is called Papeete. The current population is 283,585.

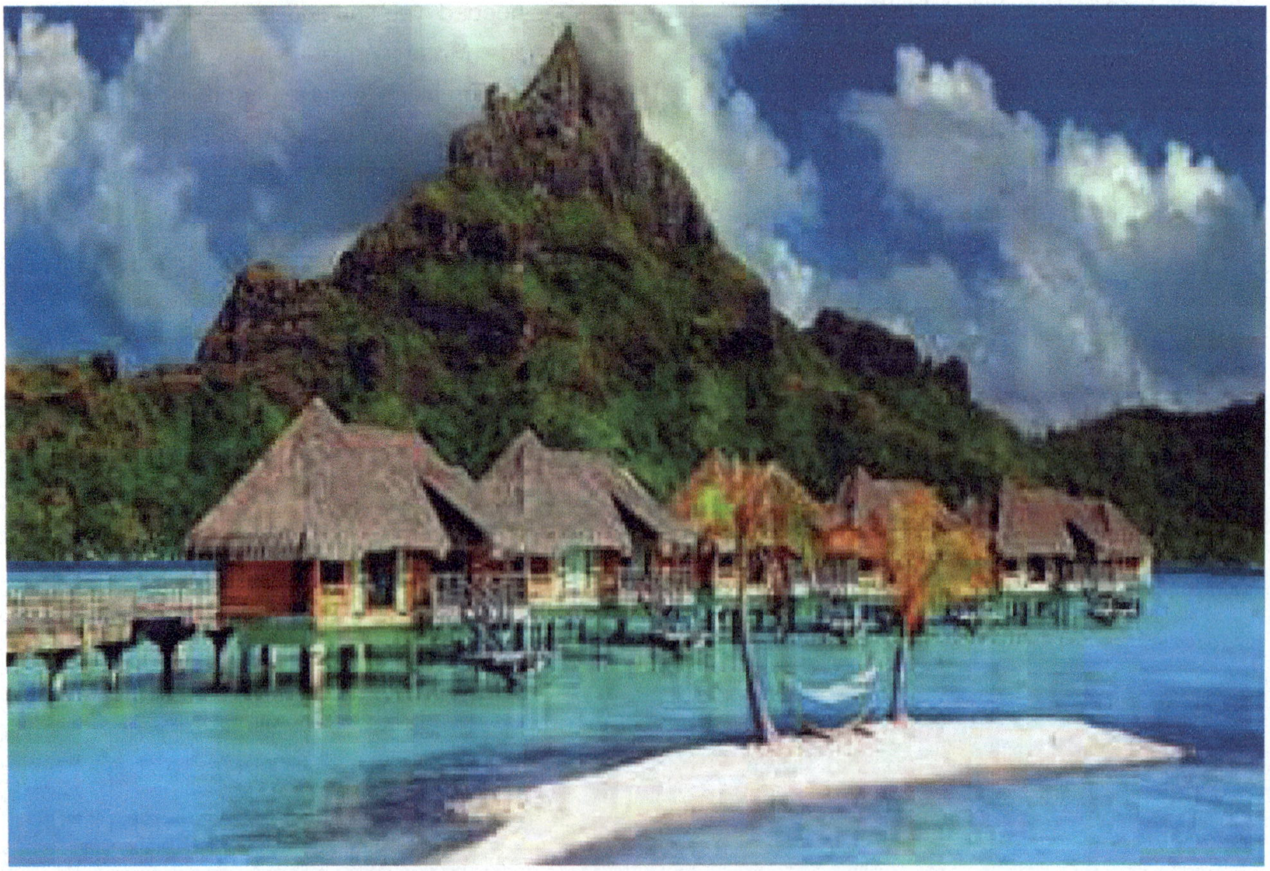

Slow-Heat French Onion Soup

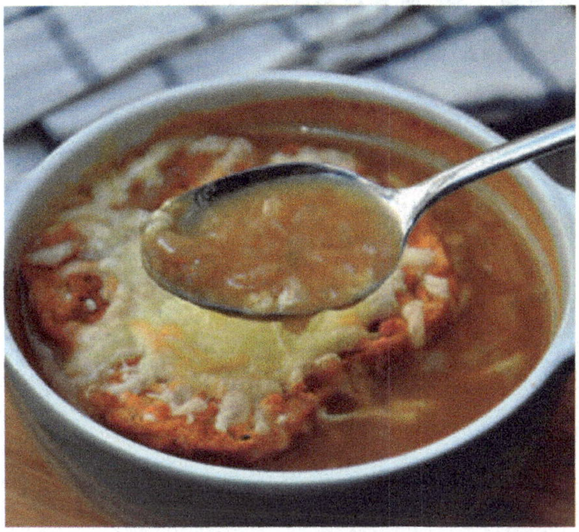

Amount of calories per serving is 147.

INGREDIENTS

- 3 large sweet onions peeled
- ⅓ cup unsalted butter
- ½ teaspoon brown sugar optional
- 8 cups beef broth 64 oz
- ⅓ cup dry white wine
- 3 sprigs fresh thyme 1 bay leaf
- ¼ teaspoon pepper
- 1 tablespoon sauce
- 1 tablespoon dry sherry optional
- 1 baguette
- 3 cups gruyere cheese
- 6 tablespoons parmesan cheese

Spicy French onion soup serves an appetizer, or a light dinner. The onion is caramelized and garnished with cheese.

DIRECTIONS

1. Slice onions ¼" thick. Cook onions, stirring occasionally, over low heat in melted butter (with sugar if using) until golden, about 30-45 minutes.
2. Add beef broth, wine, thyme, bay leaf, black pepper, Worcestershire, dry sherry. Bring to a boil, reduce heat and simmer for 1 hour. Remove bay leaf and thyme (if fresh) and discard.
3. Meanwhile, slice bread and brush with olive oil. Broil 2 minutes per side or until golden.
4. Ladle soup into ceramic bowls. Add 2 slices of bread to each bowl. Divide cheeses over bowls and broil until golden and bubbly.

THE COOK ISLANDS

The South Pacific nation with 15 islands are dispersed over a vast area.

The largest island, Rarotonga, has many epic hills.

Avarua is the national capital.

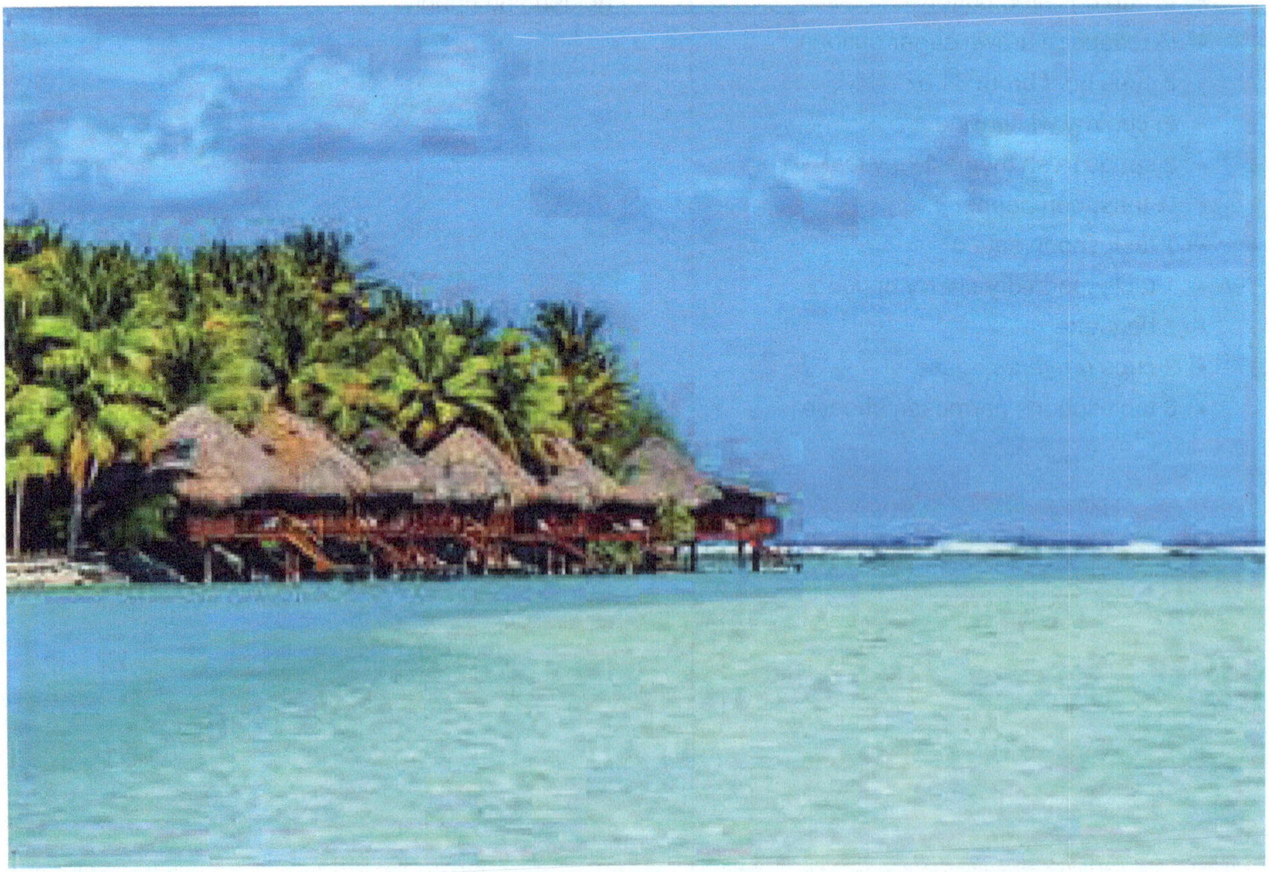

Chicken Tortilla Soup (Cook Island Style)

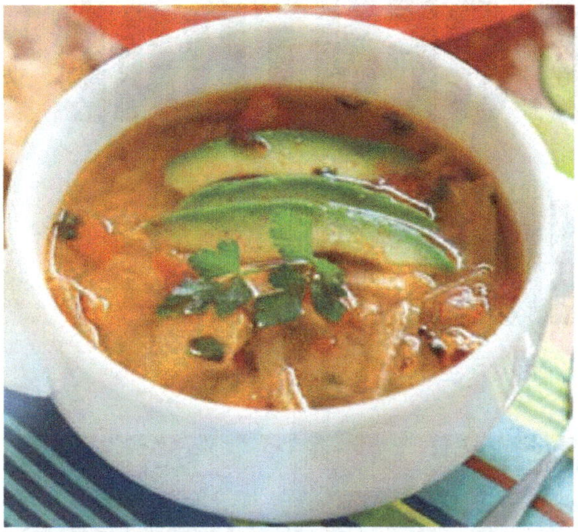

This slow-cooked protein-rich soup is a must for a complete feel of Cook Islands. It is packed full with healthy spices and will satisfy your dinner carvings.

INGREDIENTS

- 1 pound frozen chicken (shred near end of cooking time)
- 1 (15 ounce) can whole peeled tomatoes, mashed
- 1 (10 ounce) can enchilada sauce
- 1 medium onion, chopped
- 1 (4 ounce) can chopped green chili peppers
- 2 cloves garlic, minced
- 3(14.5 ounce) cans chicken broth
- 1 teaspoon cumin
- 1/4 teaspoon black pepper
- 1 (10 ounce) package frozen corn
- 1 can black beans, rinsed

DIRECTIONS

1. Place chicken, tomatoes, enchilada sauce, onion, green chiles, and garlic into a slow cooker.
2. Pour in chicken broth, and season with cumin, salt, and pepper. Stir in corn and black beans.
3. Cover and cook on Low setting for 6 to 8 hours or on High setting for 3 to 4 hours. Garnish with crushed tortilla chips, sour cream, shredded cheese, or avocados. (Note: garnishes not included in nutrition information) Makes 8 servings.

A visit to one of the sandy beaches sipping coconut water is the main gist about Cook Island.

CARIBBEAN & CENTRAL AMERICA

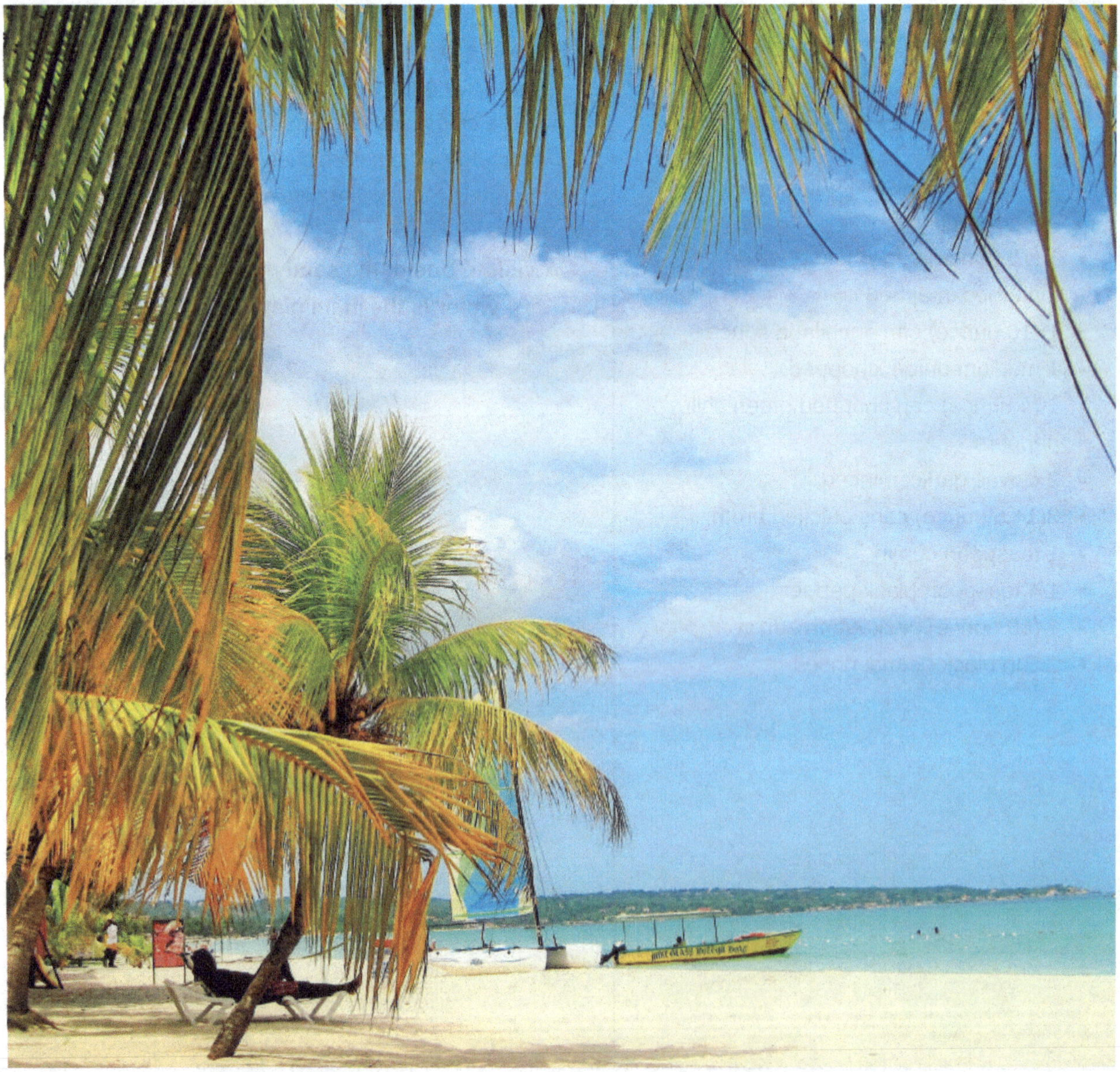

GUYANA

Guyana is also called oil-rich Guyana.

Its capital city is Georgetown.

It is culturally connected to the Caribbean through cricket, music, sports, and education.

This land of many waters has lots of virgin rainforests, and lovely waterfalls.

Guyana is also home to the one of the tallest churches – The National Cathedral at 143 feet tall, and one of longest floating bridges – Demerara harbor bridge 6,074 feet.

Guyana is known for its rich natural resources in sugar cane, rice, bauxite, gold, and diamond.

With a literacy rate of 88.5%, Guyanese are known for their educated minds and warm hospitality spirit among friends, family and tourists.

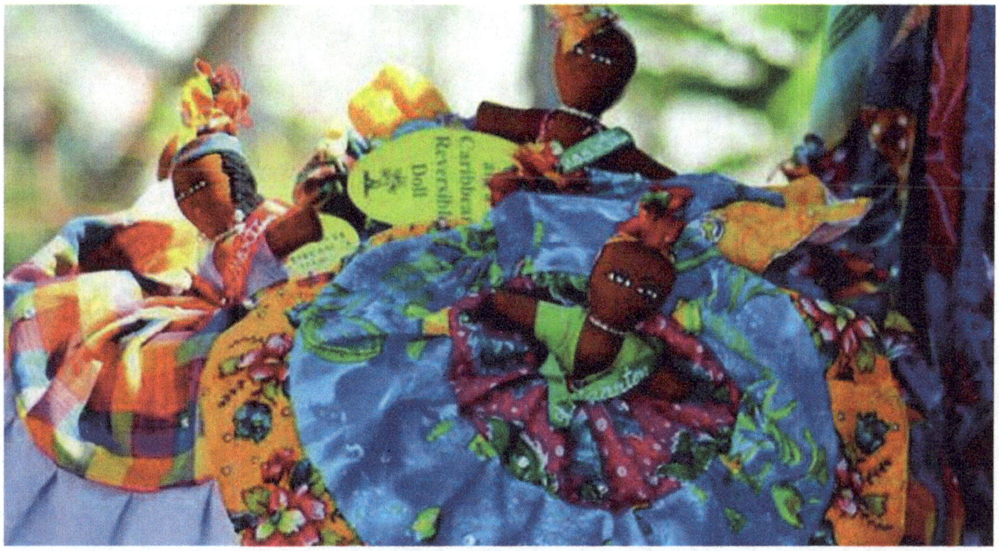

Recipe for Vegan Cornmeal Soup

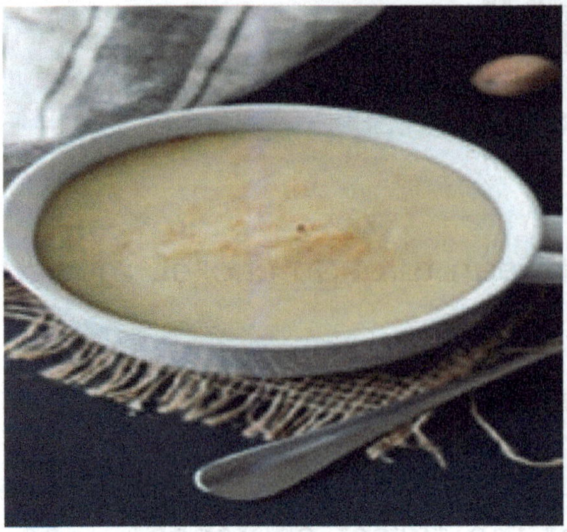

Vegan Cornmeal hearty soup is a light meal, perfect for dinner.
This is common amongst the locals in Guyana, especially in Georgetown.

INGREDIENTS

- ½ cup fine yellow cornmeal
- 3 cups water
- Pinch of salt
- 1 cup coconut milk or cream
- ¼ tsp cinnamon
- 1/8 tsp nutmeg
- ¼ tsp pure vanilla extract
- Brown sugar to taste

DIRECTIONS

1. Place cornmeal in a bowl and add 1 cup of water while stirring until smooth; set aside.
2. Place remaining 2 cups of water and salt in a pot and bring to a boil.
3. Add cornmeal and water mixture while stirring. Stir in coconut milk or cream and cinnamon.
4. Turn the heat down to a simmer and cook on low heat while stirring every 2-3 minutes.
5. After 20 minutes, stir in grated nutmeg, vanilla extract and brown sugar.
6. Remove from heat and leave to cool slightly before serving.

Guyana is quite famous for its rum as well. Come to Guyana soon. 83,000 square miles awaits you! Or Come back to Guyana soon!!

ARUBA

This South American Island capital isOranjestad.

Aruba is a generally flat, island with a population of 107,504

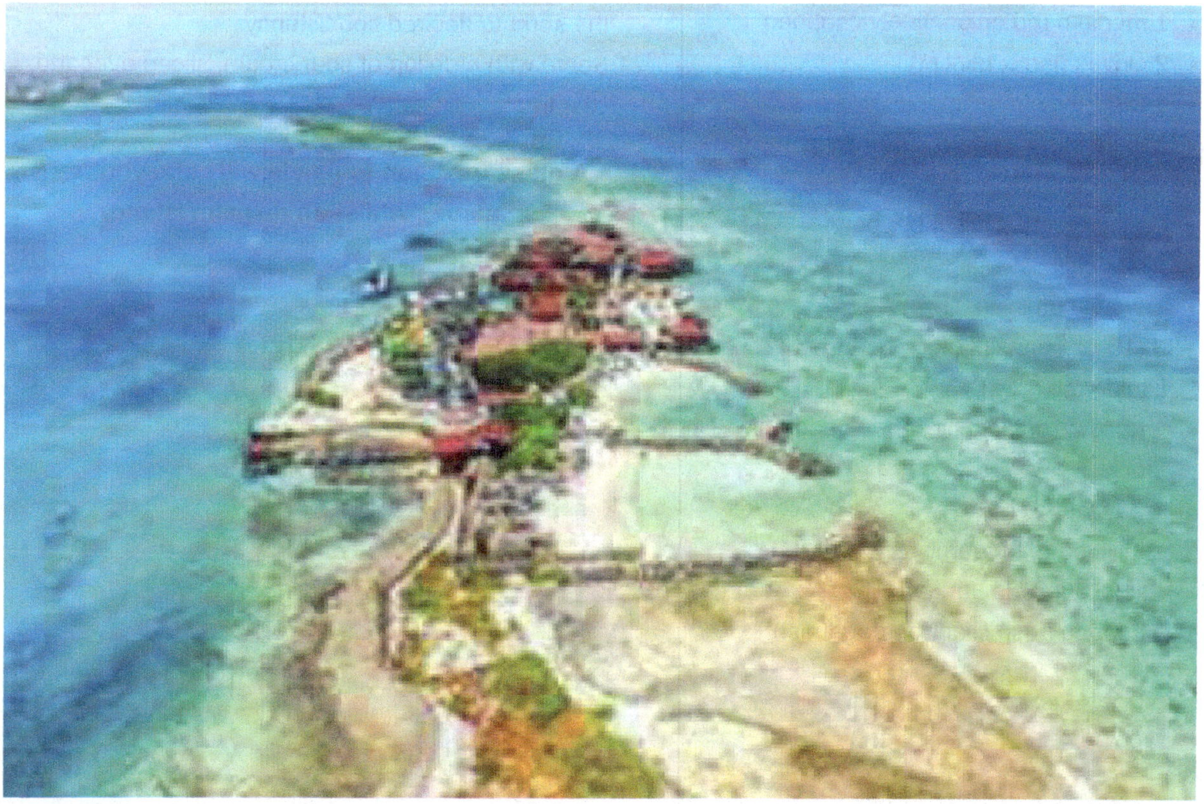

Aruban Black Bean Soup

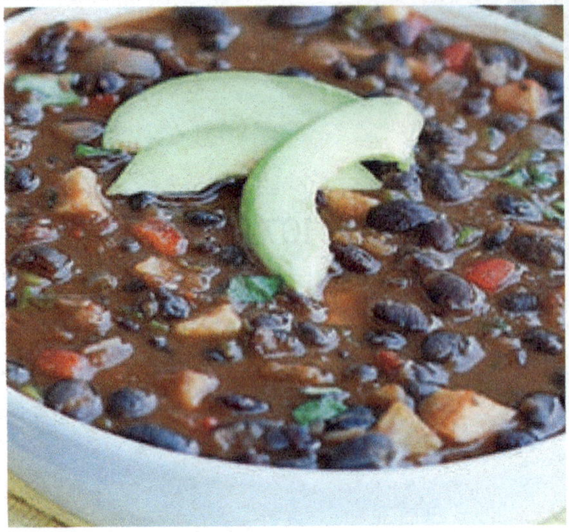

Protein-rich traditional spicy black bean soup pairs with any good Aruban drink for dinner.

INGREDIENTS

- 2 tbsp. extra-virgin olive oil
- 1 medium red onion, finely chopped
- 2 cloves garlic, minced
- 1 tbsp. minced jalapeños
- 1 tbsp. tomato paste
- kosher salt
- Freshly ground black pepper
- 1 tsp. chili powder
- 1/2 tsp. cumin
- 3 (15-oz.) cans of black beans, with liquid
- 1 qt. low-sodium chicken or vegetable stock
- 1 bay leaf
- sour cream, for garnish
- Sliced avocado, for garnish
- Chopped fresh cilantro, for garnish

DIRECTIONS

1. In a large pot over medium heat, heat oil. Add onion and cook until soft and translucent, about 5 minutes. Add jalapeños and garlic and cook until fragrant, about 2 minutes. Add tomato paste, stir to coat vegetables, and cook about a minute more. Season with salt, pepper, chili powder, and cumin and stir to coat.
2. Add black beans with their liquid and chicken broth. Stir soup, add bay leaf and bring to a boil. Immediately reduce to a simmer and let simmer until slightly reduced, about 15 minutes. Remove bay leaf.
3. Using an immersion blender or food processor, blend the soup to desired consistency.
4. Serve with a dollop of sour cream, sliced avocado, and cilantro.

A glass of Melon Popsicle will calm your tense nerves whilst on de palm Island.

SOUTH AMERICA

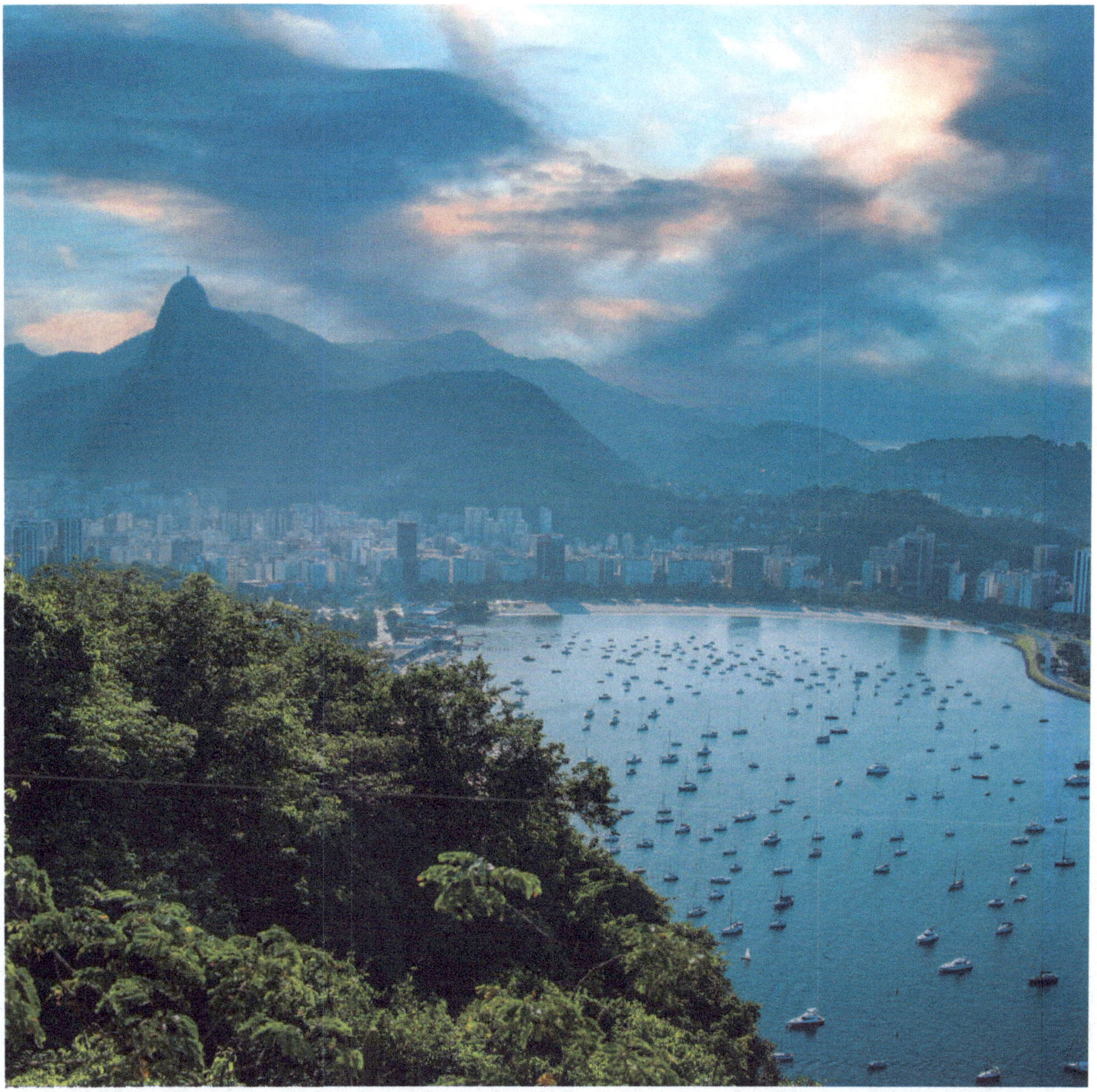

COLOMBIA

The capital of Colombia is Bogotá, and it is known for its hand to pick coffee, beautiful terrain & rich cultural heritage of music & theater.

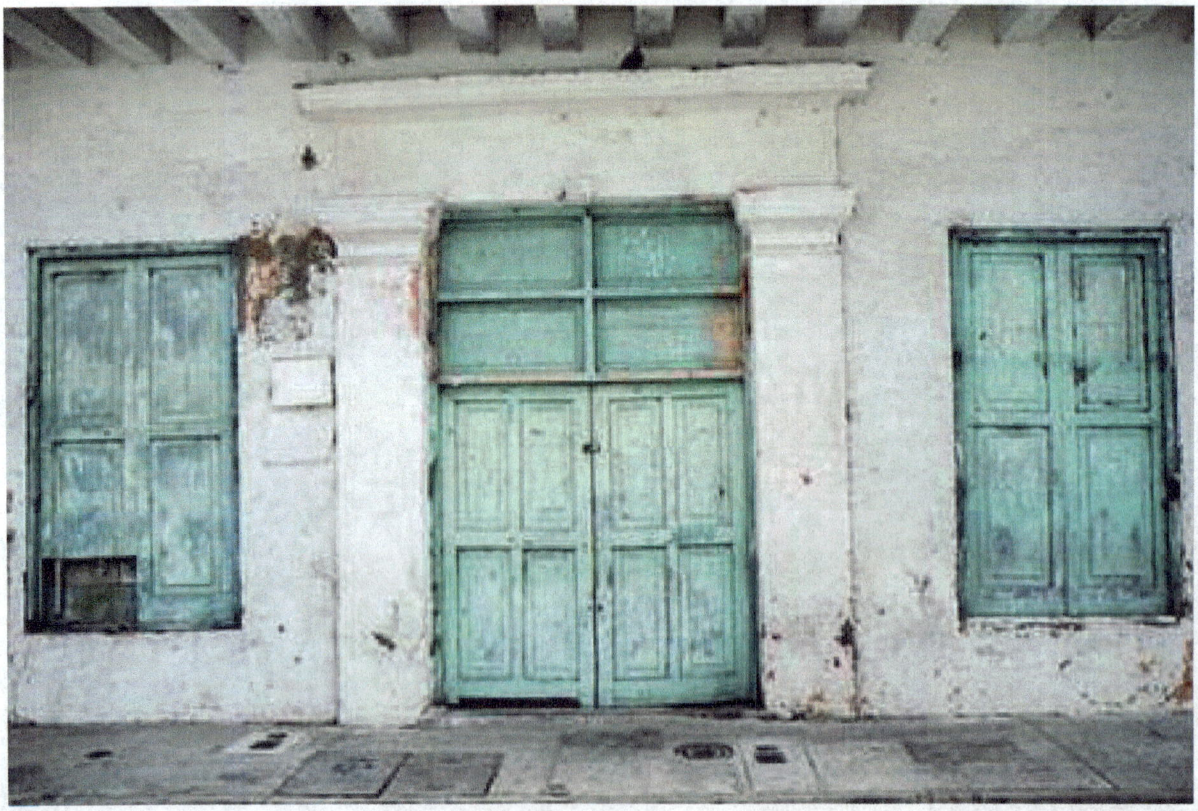

Recipe for Spanish Bean Soup

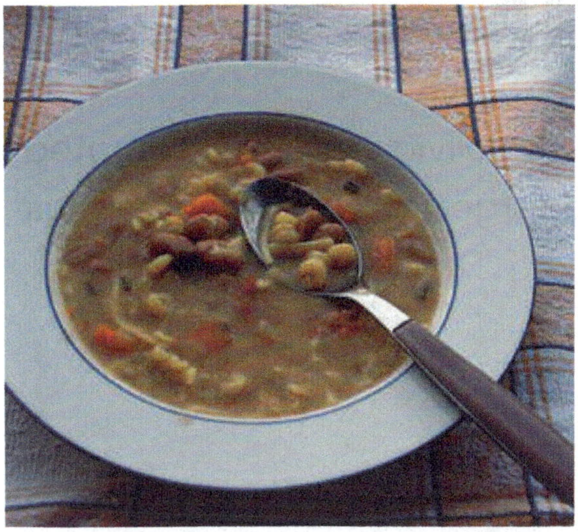

INGREDIENTS

- 1⁄2lb uncooked garbanzo bean dried (also called chickpeas)
- 1 ham bone
- 1 beef bone
- 2quarts water
- 1tablespoon salt
- 1⁄4lb salt pork cut in thin strips
- 1 onion finely chopped
- 1 chorizo sausage, sliced in thin rounds (Spanish sausage)
- 2 potatoes, peeled and cut in quarters
- 1pinch saffron
- 1⁄2teaspoon paprika

DIRECTIONS

1. Wash garbanzo beans. Soak overnight with 1 tablespoon salt in enough water to cover beans. Drain the salted water from the beans.
2. Place beans in 4-quart soup kettle; add 2 quarts of water and ham and beef bones. Cook for 45 minutes over low heat, skimming foam from the top.
3. Fry salt pork slowly in a skillet.
4. Add chopped onion and sauté lightly. Add to beans along with potatoes, paprika, and saffron. Add salt to taste.
5. When potatoes are tender, remove from heat and add chorizo. Serve hot in deep soup bowls. Serves 4.

BOLIVIA

The official capital of Bolivia is Sucre. Bolivia has an estimated population of 10.8 million persons, the largest group of indigenous people and producers of coca.

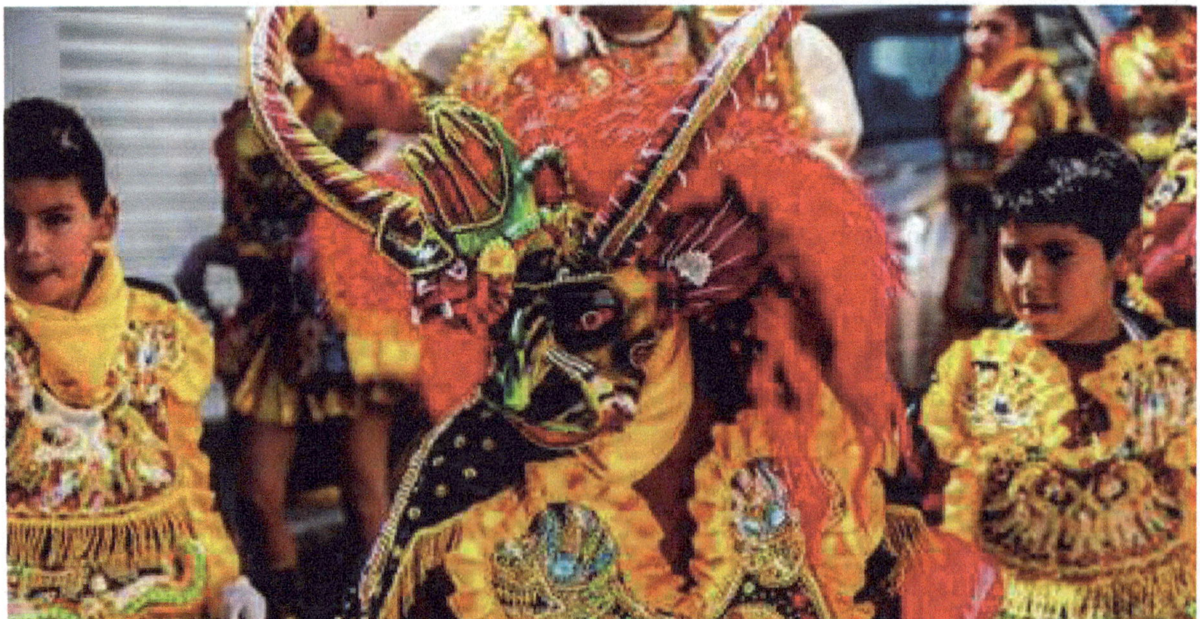

Bolivian Chicken and Noodle Soup

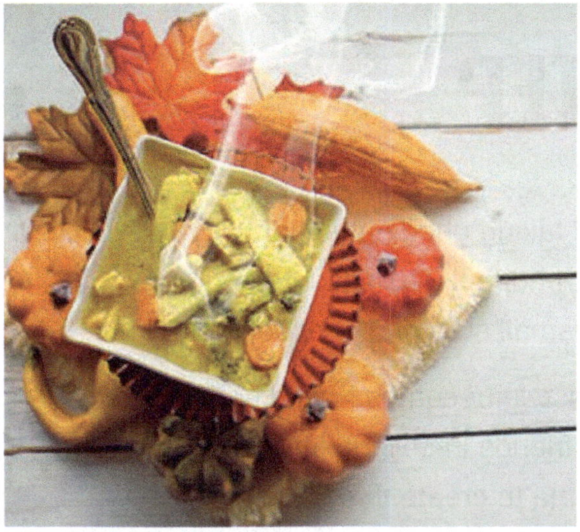

INGREDIENTS

- 1 (16 ounces) package conchiglie noodles (or your favorite noodles)
- 4 Tbsp vegetable oil
- 1 large red onion, chopped
- 1 medium bell pepper, diced
- 2 garlic cloves, minced
- 1 whole free-range chicken (about 5 pounds), rinsed, with giblets
- 4.5 quarts water
- 2 bay leaves
- 4 medium carrots, chopped
- 2 tsp pepper
- 2 tsp salt, or to taste
- 4 Tbsp fresh curled leaf parsley, chopped
- 5 ripe plantains

DIRECTIONS

1. To a large stockpot over medium heat, add oil and heat slightly. Add the noodles and fry until golden brown, stirring constantly (about 4 minutes). Remove pasta from pot with a slotted spoon and set aside.
2. To the same pot, add onions, bell peppers and garlic. Cook and stir for about 6 minutes, until the vegetables are softened and browned. Remove from the pot and set aside.
3. Place the chicken and bay leaves in the same stockpot over medium heat. Pour in 4.5 quarts of water and allow it to slowly come to a boil. Lower the heat to medium-low and gently simmer for 40 minutes - 1 hour. Carefully remove the chicken to a cutting board. When it's cool enough to handle, discard the skin, bones and giblets; shred the meat.
4. Carefully strain the stock through a fine sieve into another pot to remove any remaining solids.
5. Bring the stock, carrots and onion mixture to a gentle boil over medium heat. Cook for 5 minutes. Add pasta, salt and pepper and cook for 10 minutes, two minutes before turning it off, add chicken.
6. Sprinkle parsley before serving.
7. Serve with plantains.
8. To Cook The Plantains: Rinse and dried plantains. Cut off both ends and discard. Cut each plantain in half. Place plantains in a medium saucepan and cover with water. Bring to a boil and cook for 5 minutes. Serve hot.

NEXT STEP

Thanks for purchasing this book, reading it, and taking obedient action as you reflect on your food experiences & relationships. I hope it was enlightening and encouraging and that your life flourishes, one small step and one week at a time.

As you connect with more people & your lifestyle becomes healthier, you will influence many others around you, just like my friends in college influenced me with unique food experiences that led me to create this book.

I would love to hear from you about how this book has impacted you. Your feedback will help me in improving this book and other books in the future.

Receiving your review is important to me, it will help this book reach more people and change lives around the world.

Made in the USA
Coppell, TX
18 February 2024

29142306R00083